Good Fat is Good for Women
Menopause

Elizabeth Bright

Zenabright Press

Copyright © 2019 by Elizabeth Bright
All rights reserved. No part of this publication may be reproduced, distributed or transmitted in any form or by any means, without prior written permission.

Elizabeth Bright
Zenabright Press
Via Brigata Liguria 1
Genova, GE, 16121
www.elizabethbright.it

Publisher's Note: This is a work of nonfiction.

Cover design ©Rita Santa-Rita, www.behance.net/ritasanta-rita copyright ©2019

Good Fat is Good For Women:Menopause/Elizabeth Bright,1st ed.
ISBN 9781794665859

This book is dedicated to my daughters, Lauren and Emalia

CONTENTS

Introduction	VI
What's in a Word?	1
Menopause Is Good	35
Medicine for Menopause	44
The Case for Diet	82
Fat For Balance	116
References	151

Preface

When I first began writing this book, I realized that the women coming to my practice with symptoms of menopause were getting younger and younger. They weren't menopausal, but they did have the same symptoms attributed to menopause: weight gain, abdominal swelling, hot flashes, mood swings, chronic fatigue, problems concentrating, and vaginal dryness. I concluded that I needed to write a book about how good dietary fat—i.e., saturated fat—is essential to women of all ages, from birth to menopause.

So I changed my working title, and have made this edition the first in a series.

This makes sense to me, as a middle-aged woman, now fifty-six, looking forward and backward. I am both the mother of three children, and am myself a daughter. The way that my mother is faring in her "old age" is directly as a result of the high-carb, low-fat diet that was irresponsibly thrust upon her in her youth.

My mother was studying to be a journalist in 1956, the year representatives from the American Heart Association appeared on television to inform the American public of the "cholesterol hypothesis," advancing the theory that saturated animal and dairy fat would cause heart disease. She graduated from college with her journalism degree in 1958, the same year Ancel Keys embarked on his now debunked Seven Countries Study. My mother loved to cook, and may have bought Keys' bestselling book Eat Well and Stay Well the following year. This book was aimed at women. Women prepared the family meals, and the book instructed them to avoid saturated fat in meat and dairy and to replace animal fats with vegetable oils. The book linked saturated fat to the development of atherosclerosis, telling women that eating fat would not only cause them to get fat, but also to die of coronary heart disease. My mother is now eighty-two and struggling with Alzheimer's and osteoporosis. She is underweight, yet still worries about "getting fat." When I visited her some months ago, I saw the walking path she had beaten around her backyard. She walks so many laps, she says, because exercise will keep her healthy, even though losing her memory is so frustrating that she also tells me she wants to die.

I believe now that the depression and anxiety my two daughters faced during adolescence were influenced by my own brainwashed understanding of how to raise healthy children. After nursing for a year, I weaned them onto homemade vegetable purees and banana tofu mashes. But my homemade baby food contained no fat and not enough protein. I used to believe adolescence was inherently fraught with insecurity, but now I understand it doesn't have to be. Yes, there will always be sources of stress, but stable blood sugar levels will save teenage girls from depression and eating disorders. Like any mother, I wanted to do the best for my children, but I was misled, and it makes me angry to this day.

Although women live longer than men by almost seven years, the chances that a woman will be disabled for years before death are double those of men. What are the diseases that affect women more than men? More women die by, and seek medical care for, heart disease, stroke, fracture, osteoarthritis, obesity, diabetes, and Alzheimer's. More women than men have their thyroid removed. In the United States alone, each year approximately 600,000 women undergo hysterectomies,[1] whereas, during a ten year study from 1998 to 2011, only 962,917 men had their prostates removed.[2] More women than men have their gallbladders removed, and they often after the age of sixty; additionally, the number of cholecystectomies performed on women is increasing, while the age of female patients is decreasing. In 2011 gallbladder removal was the eighth most common operation performed in the United States. The gallbladder is necessary for the breakdown and digestion of fat. A low-fat diet interferes with gallbladder function, as it causes the liver to secrete less bile to metabolize the decreased amount of fat. The unused bile is stored in the gallbladder, where it accumulates into gallstones. When women follow the low-fat diet recommended by their doctors, those doctors then come to the conclusion that the gallbladder itself is unnecessary, even though this organ is essential for the synthesis of vitamin D.

Does being female make you more prone to disease? Certainly not. Have men also suffered from the low-fat, high-carbohydrate diet first promoted by the United States? Absolutely. But being female has been medicalized, which is the reason why, historically, more surgeries have been performed on women. As the medical historian Ornella Moscucci writes in her introduction to The Science of Woman: Gynaecology andgender in England, 1800-1929, "A deeply entrenched belief in our culture holds that sex and reproduction are more fundamental to woman's than to man's nature. Puberty, childbirth, the menopause, are deemed to affect woman's mind and body in ways which have no counterpart in man. Because of her role in reproduction, woman is regarded as a special case, a deviation from the norm represented by the male."[3]

As such, puberty, childbirth, and menopause have been treated with medication, as if they were illnesses. In women whose nutrition provides them with what their mind and body need, these stages of life pass without the sort of issues the medical industry addresses with pharmaceuticals and surgery. Unfortunately, the complications women suffer have now increased to the point of becoming an epidemic health issue, and I would argue this is because the physical and mental health of women of all ages has been damaged by low-fat diets.

In 2001, the World Health Organization calculated that the rate of chronic disease would rise by 57 percent by the year 2020.[4] That's next year. Chronic disease is no longer known as a disease of affluence, but as a disease caused by a dietary debacle: the removal of animal fat from our diet.

Animal fat was substituted with cheap vegetable oils and refined carbohydrates. The women who were alive when my mother started following US dietary guidelines to "eat healthy" and all of their daughters, all over the world, have been hurt by the vilification of saturated fat. Yes, we women want to live long lives, but more importantly, we want to live well.

Looking back, I remember the little ten-year-old who used to shout, "Sexist!" when a commercial showed a woman pouring detergent onto the collar of her husband's white shirt, before placing it lovingly into the washing machine. My mother, the woman I deeply admired for being one of the first female journalists at a major American newspaper would tell me to hush, and not be a knee-jerk feminist. But she was wrong. That little girl always wanted to save the world. This book is me trying.

Introduction

Menopause, with its hot flashes, bitchy tirades, and saggy tits, isn't something most women look forward to. Thanks to the media and the pharmaceutical industry, you may believe that your body will wither away and that your bones will crumble and your brain, which has kept you company since birth, will abandon you. But this isn't menopause. Menopause is a good thing, a deliberate evolution that only human women, orcas, and pilot whales go through. Quite the opposite of what the media sells, menopause is natural and should be an easy and harmless transition. For many women this occurs between the ages of forty-five and fifty. The idea that menopause is an "illness" is purely an invention—a sham or a condition the medical industry has forced upon women since the invention of the word "menopause" itself. You may certainly experience symptoms, but these are not due to infertility or because your period has stopped (the reasons you may have been given for your discomfort). Menopause is not to blame. The symptoms experienced are not due to a lack of estrogen, but to an imbalance in the endocrine system as a whole. This book will explain not only how these myths have been propagated and the way prescribed medical treatments can often harm menopausal women, but also how you can treat your symptoms naturally and improve your general health at the same time.

There are a lot of books about menopause. They started appearing shortly after the word was invented in 1812 (or 1821, depending upon the references you look up). These are almost all written by men who treated menopause as an illness. Some medical texts by female doctors—the first classes of women allowed to attend medical school—do mention menopause, but as a normal, natural occurrence rather than as an illness which requires treatment for symptoms with pharmaceuticals. Something natural would not require treatment.

In 1902, Dr. Emma Drake wrote that Native American and Jewish women would go through menopause without any problems and that menopause was not related to cancer, as Victorian women feared.[1] This shows us how women of different cultures can experience menopause differently. How can this be, when they were born with the same reproductive organs?

According to American physician and crusading suffragist Mary Putnam Jacobi, writing in 1895, severe symptoms during the transition into menopause were likely due to stress, malnutrition, and having children in too rapid a succession.[2] A 1926 survey of a thousand women, initiated by the *Medical Women's Federation of England and Scotland*, challenged the prevailing medical portrayal of menopause as a dangerous or significantly symptomatic event.[3]

The discovery of hormones in the early twentieth century gave rise to many more books, articles, and research papers on the subject of menopause. With the discovery of estrogen came the discovery that the level of ovarian estrogen, the first estrogen isolated, decreased with age. What would happen to women with this decline? Surely a loss of fertility must cause some sort of change in women, not just in their bodies, but also in their minds. The last fifty years have seen hundreds of works written by doctors, celebrities, celebrities with doctors, celebrity doctors, from a psychological perspective, from a fitness perspective, from spiritual and even political perspectives—all attempting to fix what isn't broken Menopause is natural, and symptoms do not occur because estrogen levels reduce with age.

In *Encounters with Aging*, which compares western and Japanese perspectives on menopause, McGill University medical anthropologist Margaret Lock writes that the reason more and more texts are being published on the subject is because baby boomers are now reaching the age of menopause.4 Her book was published in 1993. And as the women of Generation X, a smaller demographic, are now turning fifty, the texts keep coming. The new texts only differ from the old texts in how menopause is described as something requiring treatment or management. According to medical understanding, menopause today comes with a growing list of symptoms, such as Alzheimer's disease and dementia, and new drugs are still being developed to treat symptoms supposedly due to the reduced production of estrogen in the ovaries. In this book I explain that menopausal symptoms, such as the hot flash, are not due to the fact that women have a lower ovarian estrogen level.

A study in *Women in Health* found that despite the increase in articles about menopause available in the popular print media, "almost all were focused on menopause as a negative experience or disease in need of medical treatment."[5] Even though the population of the industrialized world has decreased, now that Generation X women are reaching menopause, doctors are reporting that symptoms are on the rise. There is also more confusion surrounding the safety of the treatments the medical establishment is urging on women. Aging and menopause have been joined at the hip; the word "menopause" is now interchangeable with degeneration.

Some doctors writing in the 1900s blamed menopausal symptoms on socioeconomic disparity and the new role of working women in the industrialized world.[6] More women began working long hours in dark factories. But even in our post-industrial society where many women work sedentary jobs in offices, menopausal symptoms continue to increase.[7] More and more women, among all cultures, races, and economic backgrounds, are having a harder time going through menopause. A study published in 2000 into the prevalence of menopausal symptoms in China concluded that the higher incidence of menopausal symptoms in professional women—as opposed to women in rural areas—was due to "both biological and psychosocial factors." But this doesn't tell us why women in cities reported higher rates of bone and joint disease, heart disease, and "feelings of becoming older, sad and lost."[8] Second-wave feminists blame America's youth culture for causing women to feel that age brings loss.[9] America's youth culture is not to blame for the increasing rate of menopausal symptoms in women living in Chinese cities or elsewhere across the world. America has exported something else—the high sugar diet.

It is clear that menopause and menopausal women are portrayed negatively in our society. There are many things that are wrong, and all the ways of looking at it bring up the myriad of issues women have faced, and continue to face, in our society. While this book specifically focuses on dietary and lifestyle changes, the hope is it will leave you feeling empowered, because you will have been given simple tools to help improve how you feel. The book focuses on the physical and mental changes that come with menopause, and how history and modern medicine have attempted to treat the symptoms menopause supposedly causes, and the things you can do naturally to treat your symptoms. The only side effects will be good ones, such as feeling great—probably better than you've felt since your twenties!—in a way that lasts.

Though this book is written from a female perspective, it is a collaboration between a woman and a man. I, Elizabeth, am a naturopath working in Italy, where the vast majority of my clients are women in their forties and fifties. Roderick is a naturopath working in the UK and runs a natural thyroid clinic in London. To us, this book is about more than menopause: it's about how important it is for women to have—and to maintain—a balanced endocrine system. Over the past few years, I have seen women with symptoms of endocrine imbalance getting younger, and more and more of my patients are women who in their thirties have fertility problems Their questions and the success of the treatment for which I advocate in the following chapters have inspired me to write this book. Another reason for this book is the fact that I have two daughters in their twenties, and I have seen their female friends struggling with their moods and bodies, which seem increasingly out of their control. Dr. Emma Drake wrote in 1903 that women who neglect their health when they are young are "inevitably preparing the way for a stormy menopause."[10] This book is meant to be a way to avoid that storm.

I went through menopause too. And while some of it crept up on me, the brunt of it seemed to happen overnight. To be honest, at first I was kind of excited. After all, change is cool! Menstruation had always been messy, and in my twenties, PMS often meant a week's worth of discomfort, irritability, and trips to the store for Nutter Butters. At forty-eight, I began to notice a change in my regular menstrual rhythm. Still, as will be explained later, this may have been due to other factors, because for me, menopause —or "the change," as it is sometimes rather ominously called—took me completely by surprise. My cycles became irregular. So I said, well, it's gone. Then oops, my period came back for a year, before rather emphatically going away for good. I admit I am guilty of everything this book warns against. My experience with menopause was a wake-up call, and because of it, I wish to exhort my daughters, and other women, not to do as I did.

And this is difficult! Women in their twenties don't think about the end of their fertility. Why should they? I even polled my daughters' friends and signed onto the Facebook groups they recommended, and none of these young women were thinking about menopause. This is something pharmaceutical companies are trying to change in order to create a need for pharmaceutical remedies in younger women. Advertisement for new hormone therapies are directed at women who have difficulties achieving orgasm. This is another reason I wrote this book: as a rallying cry. Not to frighten younger women, but to make it clear to them that if they avoid some of the pitfalls women have been consistently falling into over the last hundred years, they will not only have a wonderful menopause but healthy and happy years leading up to that event.

I am going to write about menopause in as much detail as possible, because the subject is still taboo enough not to be dinner-table conversation. Sex is okay to talk about; TV shows, from *Sex and the City* to *Girls*, deal with the issue of female sexuality but where are the shows that tell the stories of menopausal women? Millennials have grown up on characters like Ursula from *The Little Mermaid*, who certainly epitomizes the fat and bitchy menopausal woman. My generation had Cruella de Vil, from *One Hundred and One Dalmatians*, who was simply crazy and mean. For my mother it was the Wicked Witch of the West from *The Wizard of Oz*, who was, well, wicked. She looked older. She had a hook nose and green skin. Glinda the Good Witch of the North, with her strawberry-blond hair, shining face, and dress with white wings and low neckline, wasn't menopausal, but she would definitely be premenopausal today. In 1991, at 57, Shirley MacLaine exclaimed to *Vanity Fair*, "In Hollywood no one knows what to do with women my age."[11]

In short, I want to clear up some myths surrounding menopause to make sure you don't have a rotten time of it when it's your turn. I want to make sure that your sisters, daughters, granddaughters, cousins, friends, and friends' daughters don't either. Many women experience no symptoms during menopause, but more and more women do. Perhaps my mother never spoke to me about the symptoms of menopause because she never experienced them, or possibly because it was just not something one talked about. Often, mothers teach their daughters about menstruation simply because of the dangers of unwanted pregnancy. While puberty is a rite of passage, menopause is seen more and more as an illness that requires medication and treatment with pharmaceuticals. This is not true: menopause is not the cause of the symptoms traditionally associated with it. This book is for you whether you experience symptoms or not, and this book will help you ensure your health for the rest of your life. The decades that remain to you when you no longer menstruate should, and can be, a wonderful time of your life. This is the first time since you began menstruating that you are a female not associated with reproduction. This is a gift from Mother Nature.

CHAPTER ONE

What's in a Word?

"Given its elusiveness, perhaps menopause is not a useful term at all. It contains some meaning about which surely everyone can agree, namely that it has something to do with getting older."

—*Encounters with Aging* by Margaret Lock

"Menopause," the word itself, isn't so bad. It simply means "monthly stop." French physician Charles Pierre Louis De Gardanne came up with the term in 1812 in his book *De La Ménopause: Ou De L'âge Critique Des Femmes*—already burdening it with negativity. Or was it Charles Négrier, another French doctor writing in 1821? Whoever published it first took the roots of the word from Latin, which was itself taken from the Greek *men* meaning "moon" and *pausis*, or pause, meaning "cessation" or "stop." Something so natural has only had a name in the Western world for a little over 150 years. Etymologically speaking, "menopause" is as young as the word adolescence, but the biological function has definitely existed since time immemorial. Just like standing up and walking on two legs instead of four, menopause serves a role in beneficial evolution. But precisely because of the natural stages women pass through—puberty, pregnancy, and menopause—medicine and pharmaceutical advertising have historically targeted women for marketing and medical experimentation.

So how did we get from the literal meaning of "give me a break" to something scary that requires medical treatment, imbued with the idea of withering, insanity, and decay? When a woman goes through menopause, nothing physiological really changes other than her ability to have children. Men's reproductive capacity also declines with age, but this change isn't visible, since men do not stop menstruating, and as a result, this fact was not discovered until hormone levels could actually be measured. Women were/are identified by their reproductive capacity and, medically, identified by their reproductive organs. Menstruation meant fertility. Menstruation therefore had an inherent value for the possibility of reproduction. Ironically, bloodletting was one of the first medical treatments for menopause.

When something new is discovered in the human body its value in the body is studied, isolated, and then replicated synthetically by modern medicine. Estrogen is an example of this. Researchers will theorize situations in which a deficiency will cause problems. Humans are very resourceful, and if they can find several uses for a single discovery, its value will increase significantly. This is now called "off-label marketing." An example of this occurred when Eli Lilly and Company's patent for the antidepressant Prozac expired. They repackaged Prozac as Sarafem, garnering the seven-year right to market Sarafem to women; it claimed to treat symptoms of a new illness called Premenstrual Dysphoric Disorder. Or, in normal speak, the premenstrual blahs. One advertisement for Serafem claimed it would make women "Feel like the woman you are," because they somehow didn't already, and that this was a problem that had to be treated chemically. From surgery to hormones, the history of menopause is a medical one, foisted upon women with increasing urgency. And finding new uses for hormones doesn't stop there. The continued sexualization of women's health can now be seen in pharmaceutical companies trying to medicalize libido and orgasm.

This brings us to hormones, the "juice of life" as Suzanne Somers, actress and author of books extolling the use of "natural" hormone therapy, calls them, showing how the reproductive power of women is viewed and how women's own view of themselves can be dictated to them by advertising.

Endocrinology is a new specialty in medicine, and hormones have fascinated medical researchers since Ernest Starling discovered the first hormone, secretin, in 1902, and coined the term hormone for the chemical messengers coursing through our bodies in 1905. There are many situations in which the endocrine system might become imbalanced and may require supplementation to achieve balance. Hypothyroidism is one example of this. However, the idea that menopause is more than an imbalance is incorrect. Menopause itself, the word, and the symptoms related to the word, have been medicalized in order to create a market for replacement hormones. And women aren't the only ones to have been subjected to this phenomenon: the medical industry has created a deficiency syndrome for men as well. Erectile dysfunction is caused by an endocrine imbalance, but men take Viagra, which works mechanically, by opening and dilating blood vessels. It doesn't affect a man's biochemistry in the same way that hormones do. The fact that a woman's endocrine system involves cyclic bleeding during her reproductive years, and that it simply stops, is what makes it an easy scapegoat for the medical industry.

Aside from those women who have had hysterectomies, or in rare cases infants who are born without ovaries or other similar developmental disorders, hormone replacement chemicals have been marketed and prescribed to women to treat symptoms that were caused by other physiological processes—*not* deficiencies in estrogen or progesterone. Hormone replacement therapy has been prescribed for everything from hot flashes to aging, yet the supplementation of exogenous hormones has been linked to dangerous side effects since their creation. This has been documented before, during, and after the creation of synthetic hormones, as has the fact that the hormonal imbalance that causes the symptoms associated with menopause can be alleviated through dietary changes. But a change in diet cannot be patented. Drugs make lots more money than books about dietary change.

How did this happen? How did menopause—a natural occurrence—become a disease?

Men and Toys, from Snake Oil to Science

I originally started this chapter with the well-documented history of the medical treatment of women's diseases. Anything beyond Hippocrates's (and others') use of dietary changes often gets gruesome. From bloodletting to narcotics and poisons, to surgery the history of medicine is almost as violent as the history of disease itself. The Hippocratic principle of "first do no harm" has often been ignored in the interest of the advancement of science. The premise of this book, however, is that menopause is not a disease but a natural cessation of a physiological event, and that it exists for the benefit of women. I will, however, discuss the history of hormone therapy in this chapter, as a way to explain how diet is important to the balance of the endocrine system, and how prescribed hormones can create an imbalance and, in many situations, do more harm than good. There are certainly cases where hormone supplementation can be beneficial, but these are specific to individuals and should not be considered a blanket treatment for all women. But hormone therapy is often prescribed for all women and, disastrously, in the last two decades, for women who have not even reached menopause, as well as for young women who experience menstrual irregularities. It is a pharmaceutical tool to fix something that is not broken.

Let's look at where this all started. In the West, from ancient Greece through the Middle Ages, much of medical treatment consisted primarily of bloodletting. Hippocrates is usually credited with the idea of explaining disease as an imbalance of the humors, although his approach is similar to a traditional Chinese medical construct. His student Galen refined the idea of restoring humoral balance, often through bleeding. Certain veins were opened, such as below the nipples in women, to remove what was deemed an excess of blood to restore humoral balance. According to

Galenic doctrine, women were cold and moist, while men were hot and dry. Characteristics, temperaments, certain organs, and elements (such as fire) were associated with the four different humors. Although Hippocrates and Galen did not apply a moral judgment to either sex, they suggested a balance between male and female was best, just as we know today that some balance between sex hormones in both genders is necessary for good health in both men and women. Menstruation was healthy and natural. According to Hippocrates, women in ancient Greece went through menopause between the ages of forty-five and fifty, just as they do today.

It was Aristotle who created a hierarchy between the sexes. Men were perfect, exemplified by their dryness and heat. They were able to burn off excess toxins and, through their natural heat, maintained a healthy balance.[1] Women, however, could only eliminate toxins by bleeding. Menstrual bleeding is a function of the reproductive system, and all female diseases became associated with this. Amenorrhea, when women did not bleed, would cause toxins to rise to their head and make them insane.

In the Middle Ages, a woman who was dry and hot (like a man), had to be rendered moist and cold so that she would menstruate. The toxins that had caused this imbalance needed to be discharged through bloodletting. Although at that time amenorrhea was not connected to "a change of life" per se (the word "menopause" did not exist yet), its symptoms were similar to the symptoms that would later be associated with menopause and were caused by "being awake too much, thinking too much, being too angry or too sad, eating too little."[2] Until the invention of the word "menopause," no distinction was made between male and female aging. "Climacteric" was the word used to describe reduced reproductive capacity in both sexes. Bleeding was the treatment prescribed for most diseases. For women, this meant bloodletting from the big toe, the calves, and under the nipples.

Even though Solanus of Ephesus wrote that men and women were equal and advocated treating the whole woman, not just her reproductive organs, he believed that women suffered from illnesses particular to their sex, and was one of the first to establish a written tradition in the 1st century AD for the care of women by midwives.

In France, Louise Bourgeois (1563–1636) was instrumental in changing the perception of midwifery from the realm of folklore to science. Licensed to legally practice in 1598 and with a professional record of successful births, Bourgeois was handpicked by Queen Marie de' Medici to serve as midwife to the French royal family of King Henry IV. Bourgeois wrote several books during her retirement—the first known medical record by a woman in France—addressing childbirth, fertility, and diseases of women and infants. Later, her work was continued by Angélique du Coudray (1712–1794), who was born into a family of doctors. In a time when surgeons increasingly tried to take over medicine from women, she passed the entrance examination into the College of Surgery (École de Chirurgie). Female midwives had been barred from the college, but Du Coudray demanded that women be allowed to study at the college. It relented. She passed the entrance exam and was accepted.

In 1743, surgeons again tried to deny midwives instruction, and Du Coudray wrote a second petition, insisting that should the surgeons get their way, fewer women would receive the care they urgently needed during childbirth. At the same time, King Louis XV was attempting to address the rising infant mortality rate, and he commissioned Du Coudray to train peasant women in midwifery. Du Coudray traveled the country, teaching women her skills, and is said to have trained four thousand students directly and six thousand indirectly, as well as five hundred surgeons and physicians. She became an international symbol of France's medical progress. In addition to adding her own book of lectures to the works of Louise Bourgeois, Du Coudray invented a life-size obstetric machine to train midwives in assisting births, which was approved by the French Academy of Surgeons in 1758.

In the nineteenth century, midwives—who had been in charge of obstetrics since the time of Solanus—were pushed aside by the increasing specialization of physicians. The nineteenth century saw the creation of two new medical specialties: obstetrics and gynecology. Whereas previously menopause did not require medical attention, the newly named "condition," as of 1812 would need treatment. For nineteenth-century gynecologists and obstetricians, surgical innovations offered possibilities for career advancement and income. In France women were barred from medical schools until 1866. In England and the United States two channels of care developed, one in the United States (where women were barred from practicing midwifery) and one in England (where women were barred from medical schools until the end of the century).

Surgeons saw the financial opportunities of taking over childbirth from the domain of midwives. As Europe became industrialized, illnesses, such as cancer became more common. The original theory dating back to Hippocrates—that illness was caused by constitutional imbalance—gave way to the idea that diseases could be treated specifically where the symptom arose, such as a tumor, often through surgical intervention. With industrialization also came an increase in cancer rates, with cervical and breast cancer being the most common. The care of the female body, which had previously been the domain of midwives, became the focus of the surgeons. New techniques and surgical instruments were invented specifically for obstetrics and gynecology. The forceps, which was invented by Peter Chamberlen, a barber–surgeon, in 1588, stayed a family secret for three generations, to ensure that difficult births—for wealthy patients—were handled exclusively by Chamberlen and his descendants. Quite the antithesis to Angelique du Coudray's machine, which was freely disseminated throughout France in order to educate as many midwives as possible.[3] In modern medicine, where women were not allowed to practice (Du Coudray was an exception) commerce and medicine were linked.

Since the medical world saw that a woman's reproductive system was the source of "female" diseases, the removal of female organs became a common treatment. It was presumed that the ovaries exerted a systemic influence on women's bodies and minds, so surgeons reasoned that removing them would cure both body and mind, including menstrual problems. In 1903, Sir George H. Savage, a prominent English psychiatrist (he notably treated Virginia Woolf), said during a lecture to medical graduates, "Insanity is usually associated with the completion of the menopause."[4] By removing the ovaries, nineteenth-century surgeons believed they could treat such issues as hysteria, melancholy, nymphomania, and insanity. Thomas Schlich, a medical historian with the Max Planck Institute, describes this period as "a crucial stage in the history of modern surgery. The introduction of an ensemble of new technologies led to a new style of surgery and facilitated an unprecedented extension of the range and number of surgical interventions."[5] Since women had organs they needed only for reproduction, male surgeons were eager to experiment with new techniques on women.

Thousands of women later, oophorectomy (the current name for the removal of a woman's ovaries) was given the name Battey's Operation, after the American gynecologist who performed hundreds of such surgeries to treat menstrual disorders, epilepsy, and mania. Only one in five women survived. Critics posited that surgeons were inventing disorders in order to cure them, in a surge of commercialism that has unfortunately remained connected to menopause ever since.

Along with antivivisectionists, first-wave feminists also questioned the increasingly invasive surgical procedures practiced on women. Oophorectomies and hysterectomies became so commonplace that feminists claimed gynecologists were mutilating women with experimental operations.⁶

The first female physicians—once women were finally permitted to attend medical schools—were kinder to the idea of menopause. Before the discovery of estrogen, they wrote (as did a few their male colleagues) that menopausal symptoms were a problem in very few women, and they counseled lifestyle changes, healthy food, and in one case, fasting—perhaps harkening back to Hippocrates, who treated his patients through dietary change.⁷ These physicians—and we could say that they were a part of the first wave of feminism—tried to challenge the idea that menopause was an illness, explaining that it was rather a period when a woman could focus on herself, and even her husband, now that her children were grown. The idea that menopause needed treatment really came about with the discovery of reproductive hormones.

The Discovery of Estrogens and the Making of Synthetics

"They thought menopause. They thought menstruation. They thought beautiful skin, thicker hair, more passionate sex. They thought of curing infertility, preventing miscarriages, and drying up breast milk in mothers who preferred to bottle feed,"⁸ wrote Barbara Seaman, journalist and women's health activist, in 2003, of the possibilities doctors and pharmaceutical manufacturers believed hormone therapy offered.

Just as there have been many books written about menopause, many books have also been written about the rise of hormone therapy and how it became a hugely profitable business based on dubious claims that it could benefit women. Most importantly, these books emphasize that a natural occurrence in a woman's life became an illness so that the newly invented hormone therapies could be used to treat it. Unfortunately, this still happens in today's world, where every aspect of a woman's life is subject to her reproductive organs and her hormones.

But doctors weren't really interested in menopause; rather, a therapy that a woman could use at every stage of her life would be the most profitable treatment ever created. At the end of the 19th century things were changing: women could vote and go to medical school. Many doctors writing about menopause posited that women had menopausal symptoms because they were bored, spoiled, and wealthy—or the contrary, because they were tired from overwork and from raising large families. What kind of women had symptoms? Vain, lascivious women with loose morals who wore tight, organ-compressing corsets in order to attract the wrong kind of attention,[9] but also poor women, weakened by having many children and from working in the factory while also maintaining a family and a home. It was their own fault.

Finally, by the end of the nineteenth century, physicians, not surgeons, began rebelling against surgical procedures that sought to cure women by cutting out their reproductive organs. Sedatives that mixed opium and herbs became a popular remedy to calm the nerves. But soon doctors were experimenting with glandulars. In 1890, the German pharmaceutical giant Merck sold a popular drug called Ovarrin, which was a mixture of powdered bovine ovaries and opium.

But the thousands of women who had undergone hysterectomies and oophorectomies during those surgeries' heydey were now presenting with menopausal symptoms. Biochemists such as Sir Edward Charles Dodds, who invented the first synthetic estrogen, tried to help these women. Removing the ovaries and the uterus, producers of estrogen and progesterone, causes a great shock to the female endocrine system—a head-on collision to the delicate hormonal dance. For these women, there would be repercussions, and such repercussions would be even greater in women who were already ill, tired, overworked, and malnourished. Just as uterine, cervical, and breast cancer rates increased in the 1900s following the industrial revolution (because women worked long hours in factories and subsisted on potatoes and bread), the rate of women suffering from menopausal symptoms also increased. Researchers were still mining the female endocrine system, and perhaps if they put back what had been taken out, it would help women who had had their uterus and ovaries removed. Estrogen hormones seemed like a good answer. Adrenal hormones had not yet been discovered, and male researchers were still stopping short at the reproductive hormones; as a result, they were not connecting how the removal of the uterus and the ovaries (in order to "cure" depression, nymphomania and hysteria) affected the rest of a woman's endocrine system.

In 1928, Edgar Allen and Edward Doisy, at the Saint Louis University School of Medicine, isolated and identified estrogen. In 1928, at McGill University in Montreal, James Bertram Collip, who in 1922 produced the first insulin, synthesized from the pancreases of cows, for human beings, developed an injectable estrogen from pregnant women's urine. McGill University allowed the then-small Canadian pharmaceutical company Ayerst to market the estrogen derivative as Emminem, with Collip, the university, and the pharmaceutical company sharing royalties. Meanwhile, Edgar Allen continued his research, injecting estrogen into mice and rats. In 1941, Edgar Allen wrote an article in the journal *Cancer Research*, stating, "Estrogen is a very important factor, not merely an incidental one, in cervical carcinogenesis."[10] By this time, Ayerst had opened a subsidiary in the United States and was applying to the FDA for the approval of Emminem for the treatment of menopausal symptoms

Emminem was made from Canadian women's late-pregnancy urine, and it was expensive to produce. Ayerst first tried the urine of stallions (male urine also contains estrogen) but opted for urine from mares, as it was easier to extract. The equine estrogens were almost three times as potent as human urine. Premarin was born.

In 1929, Adolf Butenandt was also working on isolating estrogen. He was a biochemist for the German drug company Schering. Progynon was his first estrogen, also derived from the urine of pregnant women, and was sold to women to treat hot flashes and night sweats. Eventually, Butenandt and Schering also switched to horse urine and called their conjugated estrogen Progynon 2. Later, after collecting fifteen thousand liters of urine from German soldiers, Butenandt isolated progesterone in 1934 and testosterone in 1935.[11] Using prisoners from concentration camps as test subjects, Schering studied the effects of the equine hormones on his subjects, as well as other hormones developed from plants. Most of the research for estrogen therapies has been done on women who had hysterectomies and oophorectomies. Since the possible side effects of these surgeries was never considered, we'll never know if research included treatment on healthy menopausal women. The assumption was always that if estrogen was related to fertility, it could only be good for a woman in menopause.

A Nuremberg document described, "Greenhouses were built at Auschwitz to grow a rare South American plant from which female hormones could be made to lead to the sterilization of persons without their knowledge." Auschwitz survivors who knew about the experiments recounted how "women stopped menstruating and men lost their sex drive."[12] Their children of those experimented on had low IQ levels.

It was from Butenandt's work that ethinyl estradiol (EE), a synthetic steroidal estrogen, was synthesized. There are three kinds of estrogens produced in the female body, estrone (E1) which is prevalent in females before puberty and after menopause, estradiol (E2), which is the estrogen produced in the ovaries when women begin menstruating and are not pregnant, and estriol (E3), which is primarily produced during pregnancy. Ethinyl estradiol was approved for use in the United States in 1949 and is still a component in modern birth control pills. Ethinyl estradiol was originally marketed as both a contraceptive and a treatment for menopausal symptoms. However, it was eventually removed from this latter market and repackaged as a combined estrogen and progesterone because of the reports of unopposed estrogen and increased endometrial cancer. EE also has such side effects as breast tenderness, bloating, nausea, headache, and weight gain. Women who took ethinyl estradiol products also experienced a greater risk of blood clots, venous thromboembolism. Butenandt also warned about the possibility that the hormones could cause cancer.

During World War II, British biochemist Sir Edward Charles Dodds and his colleagues were in a race to beat Butenandt and Germany at the hormone game. Dodds invented a simpler non-steroidal estrogen, DES, and when he learned that Butenandt was trying to patent his creation, he published the formula for DES in *Nature* magazine in 1938. Because of the war, Dodds saw it as his duty to provide a simple, inexpensive formula for estrogen to treat the rare cases of women born without ovaries, as well as women suffering from the side effects of surgical menopause. But during the war, with most of the able-bodied men overseas, the role of women in society changed. As part of the war effort, women were working in factories as machinists, and Rosie the Riveter could do it—in more ways than one. An easy birth control method would be a timely discovery.

DES, Diethylstilbestrol, or stilbestrol as it was called in England, was cheap, easy to produce, and had the same effect as conjugated estrogens and estrogens derived from plants in that it would bind to estrogen receptors in the body. Entirely chemical, DES cost two dollars a gram, whereas urine-derived estrogen cost $300 a gram, and with DES, no horses were involved in its production. Entire books are devoted to trying to explain why the FDA felt compelled to approve DES in spite of the mounting evidence about its side effects. This was an era in love with the possibility of pharmaceutical solutions, and it wasn't until the 1970s that the huge cost of DES was understood.[13] Dodds said he never intended stilbestrol to be given to healthy women.

"Not for natural menopause, but for a woman who has had her ovaries taken out,"[14] Dodds said, when asked by Barbara Seaman how so many women suffered so many negative side effects from DES. The inventor of the first synthetic estrogen wrote that hormone drugs were very powerful and could disrupt the metabolism in every cell and organ of the body.[15]

So what was the problem with conjugated and synthetic estrogens? Estrogen promoted cell growth. Neither the conjugated estrogen nor the synthetic estrogen converted completely in the human body, and excess estrogen accumulated in tissue where there were receptors for it. It stimulated tumor growth in the breasts and uterus. All of the scientists involved saw this result in their lab tests on animals. Conjugated estrogen is several times stronger than the estrogen produced naturally by the ovaries, and the synthetic estrogen is many times stronger than that. In 1932, Antoine Lacassagne gave Butenandt's estrogen to mice and made mammary cancer. In 1939, *Journal of the American Medical Association* published an editorial against estrogen therapy, saying, "The possibility of carcinoma cannot be ignored, it appears likely that the medical profession may be importuned to prescribe patients large doses of high potency estrogens, such as stilbestrol, because of the ease of administration of these products."[16] The authors emphasized the importance of prescribing estrogen therapy for a short time and that the use should be gradually tapered off. They warned that the synthetic and conjugated estrogens should not be used as a preventative for possible menopausal symptoms in middle-aged women.

Following the drug companies' huge marketing campaign, DES was approved in 1941, although it was already clear by 1940 that DES caused cancer. Cancer researcher Dr. Michael Boris Shimkin, who later linked smoking to lung cancer, published an article in the *Journal of the National Cancer Institute* describing how DES spontaneously produced breast cancer in female mice. Apart from the fact that high doses of mare estrogen and the synthetic DES could both cause breast, uterine, and cervical cancer, it was really only the such menopausal symptoms such as hot flashes, and night sweats that these estrogens improved.[17]

But the sale of estrogen was lucrative, not just for the pharmaceutical companies but also for doctors. "I have often heard physicians say that their office expenses were paid by injections of estrogenic hormones given by their nurses."[18]

At the time, the research that demonstrated that estrogens could cause cancer had only been seen in mice and rats. Proponents of hormone therapy did not believe—or did not want to believe—that it would have the same carcinogenic effect on women. It would take two decades for reports to surface that women taking these estrogens were getting cancer.

Biochemists had worked feverishly to isolate reproductive hormones, and the 1950s pharmaceutical companies in Canada, the US, and Germany were creating huge campaigns to market their products to menopausal women. Surgeons had marketed hysterectomies and oophorectomies in the nineteenth century when industrial England saw a surge in cervical cancer.[19] Cancer was seen as a stigma, and was already discussed as a genetic trait. Women had preventative surgery to ensure they did not get it—just as woman today sometimes have mastectomies if they have a gene that is reportedly supposed to predispose them to breast cancer. Just as invasive and ineffective surgeries became a societal obligation for women, marketing menopause as a deficiency created a market for new products. Since estrogen was linked to fertility, menopause, by consequence, meant women were deficient in it. Estrogen was isolated, but it was not yet measured. Since fertility meant, to men, health and beauty, a decline in the hormone that signified fertility would hasten the arrival of all the physical changes associated with aging. They did not yet understand that other organs and peripheral tissue take over the production of estrogen during menopause. This was not discovered until 1988.

Since medicine had always associated a woman's illness with her reproductive system, medical researchers did not look further than the decline in estrogen to explain menopausal symptoms. In 1939, J. P. Pratt, the chief of gynecology and obstetrics for the acclaimed Henry Ford Hospital in Detroit, wrote that with all the symptoms blamed on menopause "would not be complete unless nearly all the index in a textbook of medicine were included."[20] It seemed as if doctors were blaming any symptom a woman who naturally stopped menstruating could have on menopause.

Suddenly gynecologists had a new variation on the shiny new surgical tool. DES could be purified and standardized more easily than estrogens derived from horse urine and could be taken in pill form, which meant gynecologists could treat dozens of women a day. Whereas the original version of conjugated estrogen could only be administered in the form of painful injections, now all they needed to do was write a prescription. Despite the reports of cancer, hormone therapy was new and backed by a huge marketing campaign; even those doctors who were not directly financed by the hormone manufacturers would have found it difficult not to emulate their peers. This was modern medicine, believed to be infallible. Though the biochemists urged caution, the doctors had women in their offices with symptoms. As women who did not have symptoms did not go to the doctors, the doctors' perception of how menopause affected women became skewed. These doctors then convinced the FDA of the efficacy and safety of estrogen hormone treatment for menopausal symptoms.

There were doctors who advised caution, however. In his article "The Management of the Menopause" for the *American Journal of Obstetrics and Gynecology* in 1940, Dr. Emil Novak wrote that the symptoms of menopause were "explainable more rationally as the result of the stress and strain resulting from the rearing of large families of children, or because of domestic, economic, or marital problems";[21] note that this is the same argument the doctors opposed to "oophorectomies and hysterectomies made before the discovery of estrogen.

In 1941, the US Food and Drug Administration approved the sale and prescription of DES for symptoms of menopause. Soon it was prescribed for a variety of different conditions. Gynecologist Karl John Karnaky, who ran a private clinic in Texas, injected huge amounts of DES into the wombs of pregnant women to prevent miscarriage. This had never been approved. It was also prescribed as hormone replacement therapy for such conditions as breast and prostate cancer, premenstrual syndrome, acne, stopping lactation, and to slow the growth of girls who "were at risk for getting too tall."[22] All of this despite the fact that DES had not been proven to have any beneficial effects beyond improving hot flashes associated with menopause specifically in women who'd undergone surgical menopause. According to Nancy Langston in her book *Toxic Bodies: Hormone Disruptors and the Legacy of DES*, many women were not even informed that they were taking a synthetic hormone.

Only two years after its development, it was documented that as many as 80 percent of women prescribed DES experienced nausea and vomiting. Even though nausea and vomiting are toxic reactions, because these were symptoms already associated with menopause, researchers decided that DES was not the cause. Two investigating physicians even went so far as to claim that patients suffering from nausea and vomiting while on DES were neurotic. From 1941 to 1971, doctors prescribed DES to millions of women, initially for menopause and then to prevent miscarriage. Besides nausea and vomiting, it also had the immediate side effects of bloating and dizziness and the long-term side effects of liver damage and cancer. It also disrupted sexual development. In 1971, DES was shown to cause vaginal tumors in females who had been exposed to the synthetic hormone in utero. The FDA immediately recommended against prescribing DES to pregnant women, but the drug was not banned.

Although warning labels were slapped onto the packaging—as was eventually done with cigarette packs—doctors in the US were still prescribing DES as birth control as recently as the 1980s. Over 200 drug companies produced DES worldwide. Internationally, this went on even longer. The DES daughters—women who developed cancer after being exposed to DES in utero—brought a huge lawsuit against several drug companies, including Eli Lilly and as a result, today's pharmaceutical companies are forced to list possible side effects in their advertisements.

In her study of the DES case, Nancy Langston writes that the FDA "chose the health of big business over public good," and that the pharmaceutical companies "skillfully manipulated scientific uncertainty to delay regulation."[23]

In 1953, Schering pharmaceuticals (now Bayer Schering Pharma AG) released a video to "educate" physicians and promote ethinyl estradiol therapy—which is still the major component in contraceptives today. It opens to a matronly woman, somewhere in the country, taking in laundry from the backyard, while the male voiceover states that declining reproductive capacity only happens to women. This "country woman," we presume, is eating a healthy diet and breathing fresh country air and is engaged only in "housework." Just as the voiceover has finished saying, "While the majority of women pass through this change without problems," [women in the country] the film cuts to a busy doctor's office where several smartly dressed younger women wait their turn. The voiceover explains their presence by saying, "The menopause can bring symptoms so disturbing that medical help must be sought," and that "this can occur as young as 35."

The symptoms described are not only the usual vasomotor symptoms of hot flashes and night sweats, but also "deep depression, loss of sense of well-being, indifference to surroundings." The voiceover explains that these women —the smartly dressed ones in the doctor's office—need psychotherapy, sedatives, and ethinyl estradiol. Other symptoms are "diffuse aches and pains, insomnia, gastrointestinal disturbances, and loss of libido," the man's voice explains. The final image is of a doctor writing a prescription for ethinyl estradiol, as the voiceover concludes, "Woman's menopausal symptoms are caused by her emotional fragility, and can only be helped, *must* be helped by sedatives and estrogens."

By 1960, there were reports that 60 to 90 percent of women exposed to DES in utero were born with abnormal sex organs. High rates of infertility, miscarriages, and cervical cancer were documented. DES sons were born with testicular dysfunction and were often sterile. DES mothers, as they came to call themselves, had a 40 percent increase of breast cancer. After 1975, DES was no longer recommended for any therapy except as an anti-androgen for prostate cancer, though Eli Lilly continued to produce and market it until 1997.

Sales for DES peaked in the 1950s, and no clinical trials ever proved its effectiveness for the conditions for which it was so often, tragically, prescribed. Although it is still prescribed for advanced prostate cancer and some cases of metastatic breast cancer, doctors treating menopause turned to Premarin, the conjugated estrogen derived from horse urine.

Psychiatry

Amazingly, hormone therapy fell somewhat out of favor after World War II. The double whammy of insanity and depression aimed at women and their declining hormones moved instead to the Freudian couch.

In the Victorian era, menopause was associated with sin and decay, which informed even influential women psychiatrists who perpetuated the idea that menopause was a period of decline. In 1924, Helene Deutsch became the first female psychoanalyst to write about menopause.[24] She followed the traditional Freudian model, which held that menopausal symptoms were related to a decline in libido. Deutsch wrote that symptoms of menopause, such as anxiety, palpitations, and high pulse rates, were caused by this decline in libido and the "devaluation of the genitals as an organ of reproduction." She followed her mentor Freud's conclusion that menopause was psychologically troubling to women, that it created neuroses and anxiety, and that it would turn into a physical illness. Freud himself wrote that "after women have abandoned their genital functions" "They, [women] become quarrelsome, peevish, and argumentative, petty and miserly, in fact, they display sadistic and anal-erotic traits which were not there in the era of womanliness."[25] We see this model echoed in later advertisements for hormone treatments, which, during the 1940s and 1950s, suggested it was a woman's responsibility to take hormone treatments so as not to burden her family with her changes in mood.

Although psychoanalysis eventually evolved from the strict model of basing a woman's mental state on her psychosexual development, both psychology and psychiatry have focused on treating menopause as a self-esteem issue, presuming that a menopausal woman becomes depressed because she can no longer fulfill her purpose of having children or because she has lost the youth that made her attractive. A later development included hormonal changes that supposedly contributed to the desexualization of women. One female psychologist even wrote that menopause "adds only one factor: it diminishes that part of the integrative strength of the personality which is dependent upon the stimulation by gonadal hormones."[26]

After only a decade, the boom in psychotherapy declined in the United States. The treatment seemed only to explain problems, giving them Freudian names (see above anal-erotic sadism for menopause), rather than fixing them. In 1952, psychologist Hans Eysenck wrote in an article that his patients' conditions were about as likely to improve whether they received psychotherapy or not, and that many simply got better on their own.[27] In the modern climate of medical science, surely a pill could do better for this new disease of "menopause."

Premarin

The historical perception of menopause started off as a divide. Many doctors saw it as a natural transition for women and gave great importance to a woman's general health as a deciding factor in the development of menopausal symptoms. But the story of how conjugated estrogen, ethinyl estradiol, and diethylstilbestrol came to be approved shows how commerce was a driving force in the medicalization of menopause. Drug companies implemented the language of loss, which is the language of deficiency, of the loss of youth and of sexuality, became associated with menopause.[28]

In 1943, Ayerst, the makers of Premarin, merged with Wyeth. Wyeth-Ayerst could therefore provide both "sythentic" estrogen (DES) and a "natural" estrogen (Premarin). An advertisement for Wyeth Estrogens in the *American Journal of Obstetrics and Gynecology* at the time touted both estrogens for "When the ovary goes into Retirement," depicting a despairing woman in her thirties sitting in an armchair, cradling her head in her hand. At the same time as the first synthetic hormone replacement therapy went on the market, modern medicine was surreptitiously convincing women that they needed to prepare for debilitating symptoms and possibly life-threatening health risks once they reached the age of menopause.

Robert B. Greenblatt was a pioneer in reproductive endocrinology—a new medical field that developed after World War II. He developed the testosterone pellet, which he used to treat women with gynecological disorders and which required surgical implantation. Women came to his private studio from all over the world. Sometimes he treated more than thirty women a day with hormones. He believed wholeheartedly in the efficacy of hormone replacement therapy and viewed menopause as a deficiency disease, a condition in need of treatment. "All menopause is divided into three kinds of miseries, he said."[29] The first misery included hot flashes, sweats, palpitations, spasms, and the sensation of a lump in the throat of the kind related to hysteria. The second misery consisted of mood disturbances, such as depression, anxiety, and insomnia. The third misery was metabolic dysfunction. Even though doctors such as J.P. Pratt warned in 1939 that too many of women's health issues were being treated with hormones, it did not occur to Greenblatt that women might have other issues not necessarily related to sex hormones.

In her book *The Estrogen Elixir*, Elizabeth Siegel Watkins describes how, before the 1960s, doctors treated menopause with a three-part protocol. First, they treated women with menopausal issues with counseling, then sedatives, and then finally hormone therapy. But companies engaged in aggressive advertising to change that. As we've seen, advertisements in the 1940s already depicted women as unstable. Premarin was the first to suggest that hormone therapy could help stabilize women's moods. "An increasing number of investigators are commenting on the 'general sense of well-being,' which is usually experienced by menopausal patients following Premarin administration," one advertisement claimed. Hormone therapy wasn't only good for relieving women of physical symptoms, but it could also make them happy!

Wyeth-Ayerst was not alone in this. Abbot, another pharmaceutical company selling hormone therapy, showed an image of an older woman weeping over a picture of her younger self. "Arrival of the menopause need not cause a woman to feel that she must face a future devoid of femininity and charm," reads the caption. One ad even depicted Mrs. Jekyll and Mrs. Hyde. On estrogen therapy, Mrs. Hyde would no longer turn into Mrs. Jekyll. Menopause became "the menopause syndrome," and with it a woman's connection to her fertile life was severed, which put her in need of estrogen replacement therapy. Since the ads depicted younger women, and proclaimed that estrogen would help women "enjoy their forties," it becomes clear that hormone manufacturers were attempting to convince women they needed treatment long before they reached menopause.

Through ad campaigns, Ayerst successfully made the more expensive Premarin the most prescribed estrogen for hormone therapy in North America—even when it became evident that after the first year of using Premarin, one in ten women developed endometrial growth that could become malignant. After the third year of Premarin therapy, the risk rose to one in three. But these were older women. Perhaps it was age, some doctors reasoned—women weren't supposed to live past menopause anyway. Modern medicine had lengthened a woman's lifespan, they contended. And anyway, there had been no long-term trials of estrogens on humans.

Premarin cost more. The advertising campaign depicted stylish, swanky women in sailboats. They'd found the fountain of youth and often stood draped on the arm of handsome, well-dressed husbands, who looked at them adoringly. But the ads also had a pernicious way of suggesting it was a woman's wifely duty to take Premarin. One colorful advertisement, featuring an attractive and wealthy couple on a sailboat, reads, "The physician who puts a woman on 'Premarin' when she is suffering in the menopause usually makes her pleasant to live with once again. It is no easy thing to take the stings and barbs of business life, then to come home to the turmoil of a woman 'going through the change in her life.'"[30]

Marketing began to imply that hormone replacement therapy (HRT) was a way to keep women young and their moods balanced. If youth and fertility were associated with estrogen production, it was easy for advertising companies to switch horses, from selling estrogen to treat menopause symptoms to marketing it as an elixir of youth.

In his book *Feminine Forever*, Brooklyn gynecologist Robert Wilson argued that the menopausal woman was "an unstable estrogen starved" woman, who is responsible for "untold misery of alcoholism, drug addiction, divorce and broken homes."

This book was a bestseller. A menopausal woman was suffering from a deficiency, which would make her wither. With HRT, "her skin becomes subtle again, the muscles regain their tone and strength, the breasts are restored to their former fullness and contours, the genitals again become supple and distensible, skin cracks and genital inflammation heals. Bones that have become brittle regain most of their former strength." By taking synthetic estrogens she could remain "feminine," which undoubtedly meant looking as if she could be reproductive—or else, what would be the point?[30]

Published in 1966, Wilson's was the first book to promote estrogen therapy. While doctors had initially started prescribing estrogen therapy for hot flashes, both DES and Premarin and other estrogen preparations had been prescribed for infertility and miscarriages. Now here was a gynecologist who promoted estrogen not only as a fountain of youth, but also as a way to prevent age-related illnesses, from breast cancer (yes even cancer) to osteoporosis.

Vogue introduced Robert Wilson as a "famous and distinguished gynecologist" and in one issue of the magazine included an abridged version of his book. It was everywhere. Eventually it was reported that Robert Wilson had received thousands of dollars from drug companies selling hormone therapy, including Wyeth-Ayerst, the makers of

Premarin. Wyeth-Ayerst launched campaigns directed at doctors, spearheading one of the greatest advertising campaigns of the time. Promotional material found its way into doctors' offices; women's magazines published not only articles but also glossy ads, which became more and more misogynistic. Women with ovaries that no longer produced estrogen would suffer decades of deficiency; those who took Premarin were depicted as young and sexy, while those who did not became old, wrinkled, and stooped. In 1963, with funding from pharmaceutical companies, Robert Wilson founded the Wilson Research Foundation, whose manifesto was to educate the medical community and the public about HRT to further push the marketing of various estrogens. According to Wilson, any illness, any difficulty, both mental and physical, could be blamed on a lack of estrogen. He promoted long-term estrogen treatment, which, as we have seen, scientists advised against.

In 1969 his best-selling book, *Everything You Ever Wanted To Know About Sex: But Were Afraid to Ask*, David Reuben described the menopausal woman this way:

"When a woman sees her womanly attributes disappearing before her eyes, she is bound to get a little depressed and irritable. . . . Having outlived their ovaries, they may have outlived their usefulness as human beings. The remaining years may be just marking time until they follow their glands into oblivion."[31]

Some doctors and magazine editors did try to stop the flood. One writer in *Better Homes and Gardens*, one of the most widely read women's magazines at the time, wrote, "Menopause does not produce chronic degenerative diseases such as cancer, heart disorders, and arthritis."[32] But Wilson's book, *Feminine Forever*, caused Premarin sales to triple. They remained record-breaking until the mid 1970s.

In the early 1970s, second-wave feminists started reacting to the defeminizing and misogynistic caricatures of middle-aged and older women. The docile, sedated, and handled woman, who existed only to keep house, bear children, and then keep house and husband happy, was not accepted by liberated women. Germaine Greer, writer and feminist activist, famously addressed a convention of gynecologists with, "Gentleman, you see before you a noncompliant woman."[33] Feminists argued that medicine, because of their natural bodily experiences such as menstruation and childbirth, had marginalized women.

As a result, drug companies changed tactics. They co-opted medical language and came up with a new ad campaign that moved away from menopausal women's subjective symptoms to medical evidence. Ads now came displayed graphs, X-rays, and images of osteoporotic bones. Formatrix was born, a combination of Premarin and testosterone that included vitamin C for good measure. Sales of Premarin had dipped in the 1970s, but with this new advertising campaign offering a medical message, sales soared again. By the 1990s, heart disease and Alzheimer's were added to the list of diseases hormone replacement therapy, in the form of conjugated estrogen, could prevent and possibly cure. From a temporary treatment for hot flashes for the 10 percent of women who reported menopausal symptoms in the 1940s, to the fountain of youth for middle-aged women in the 1960s, to the emancipated women of the 1970s, estrogen therapy became essential for a healthy lifestyle.

Wyeth-Ayerst,"displayed a remarkable ability to refashion the product, adapting it to changing scientific evidence, social and political contexts, and regulatory environments," wrote the historian Alison Li.[34] Premarin became the fifth most prescribed pharmaceutical in the United States during this time. In the 1990s, Premarin became the number one dispensed drug in the United States, even though in 1982 cancer research reported that conjugated estrogen therapies were a major factor in the development of cancer in women. Boston University Medical Center published research that hormone therapy was the cause of more than 15,000 cases of endometrial cancer in the United States between 1971 and 1975 alone. The report stated that hormone therapy caused the largest iatrogenic disease (disease caused by doctor-prescribed treatment) in the history of the United States.

Because of reports such as these, the Women's Health Initiative was launched. Clinical trials were designed to get to the bottom of over sixty years of health claims by pharmaceutical companies to conclude whether hormonal therapy or diet modification, and supplements such as vitamin D and calcium had a beneficial effect on heart disease, bone density, and colorectal cancer. These trials would take years. In the meantime, Wyeth-Ayerst added Progestin to estrogen hormone therapy to counteract the stimulated growth of cancer cells in women who took hormone therapy. Prempro was approved by the FDA in 1995, even though a Swedish study had shown that women on both combined estrogen and progestin therapy were actually at double the risk of breast cancer. Wyeth had ghostwriters flood magazines and medical journals with articles that downplayed the risks and implied unproven benefits—like protection from dementia and even enhanced eyesight, better skin, and augmented self-esteem. For example, Dr. Wulf Utian, a South African gynecologist, was to view menopause as a health related-issue during a visit to a pharmaceutical company in West Berlin in 1967. On Wikipedia he is quoted as saying, "A new female hormone was mentioned and thereby started my interest in the subject. Upon my return [home] I approached the Chairman of the Department of Gynaecology of the University of Cape Town ... and spelled out my plans for a menopause clinic." [35]

Utian wrote *The Menopause Manual* in 1978, and *Managing your Menopause* in 1990. He founded the International Menopause Society and the National Menopause Society of the United States. In 2002, on CBS News, after the WHI debacle, he was made to admit that he received financial support from Premarin's manufacturers. With Utian's help and the help of other physicians promoting hormone therapy, Premarin sales reached one billion dollars in 1997.

To further increase sales, Wyeth hired DesignWrite to write articles and manuscripts about Premarin's supposed health benefits for publication in medical journals. According to a proposal the company submitted to Wyeth, these publications would serve to "increase physician awareness on the multitude of benefits that hormone replacement therapy provides" and "diminish the negative perceptions associated with estrogens and cancer."[36]

The US government abruptly halted the huge Women's Health Institute's study in 2001, deciding it was too dangerous to continue. The trial studied 16,608 women, but those who were taking a combination of estrogen and progestin hormones had more instances of breast cancer, more heart attacks, more strokes, more pulmonary embolisms, and more blood clots than the women taking a placebo. More studies in 2003 reiterated the findings from 2001. After the announcement of the trial results, Prempro sales plummeted by 32 percent. Wyeth-Ayerst's (now Pfizer's) stock prices fell by 19 percent. As evidence kept mounting, the FDA ordered both Premarin and Prempro packages to include warning labels stating that, by taking them, women were at increased risk of heart disease, stroke, breast cancer, pulmonary embolisms, and blood clots.

Wyeth-Ayerst, which became Pfizer, is still being investigated for the way in which it managed to convince doctors and millions of women that conjugated estrogens were actually beneficial. What started as a treatment for hot flashes associated with declining ovarian estrogen production became preventative care against illnesses associated with aging. It was no longer enough to take conjugated estrogens after reaching menopause; to ensure optimum health, women needed to take the hormones before and after.

Many lawsuits have been filed against Wyeth, and billions of dollars have been paid in damages. In 2009, the *New York Times* published an article titled "Menopause, as Brought to You by Big Pharma." The article quotes Dr. Avorn, a professor of medicine at Harvard University, who wrote an article on the subject for the *Journal of the American Medical Association* as saying, "The information coming out in litigation helps us understand how a belief in a 'protective benefit' of estrogens on the heart was able to spread like wildfire through the medical community."[37]

Bio Identical Hormones

Bio-identical hormones, called BHRT, derived from soybeans or yams, soon became an alternative to equine estrogens. A "bio-identical hormone" is defined as a molecule structurally identical to the progesterone produced by a woman's body. John R. Lee, in his 1995 book *Natural Progesterone: The Multiple Roles of a Remarkable Hormone*, criticized conjugated estrogen theory and promoted the therapeutic use of natural progesterone to treat menopausal symptoms, including the age-related illnesses estrogen had been purported to address, such as osteoporosis and heart disease. John R. Lee, with Jonathan Wright, pioneered the use of BHRT in order to alleviate estrogen dominance, which Lee argued was the cause of menopausal symptoms. With so many women on estrogen therapy, this seems plausible. But estrogen dominance is also a result of a high carbohydrate diet

Most medical organizations, such as the North American Menopause Society—whose founding executive director, Dr. Wulf Utian, received financial support from the manufacturers of Premarin—released statements that Lee's claims were unproven, and critics pointed out that bio-identical hormone therapy, which was derived from plants, was not any more natural than equine estrogens. derived from the many horses destroyed in the production of Premarin. However most of the powerful conjugated equine estrogens extracted from pregnant horse urine do not convert to human estrogens once they enter the body. This can cause dangerous amounts of cancer-causing unopposed estrogens to accumulate in tissues. According to the proponents of bio-identical hormones, the amount of equine estrogen that does not convert to human estrogen is the cause of the dangerous side effects, such as cancers when estrogen is in excess.

Suzanne Somers wrote her bestselling book *The Sexy Years: Discover the Hormone Connection* in 2004. In it she described that getting older had been "brutal" for her, and that she had banished the "Seven Dwarfs of Menopause"—Itchy, Bitchy, Sweaty, Sleepy, Bloated, Forgetful, and All-Dried-Up—by taking bio-identical hormones. Since hormone replacement therapy came with dangerous side effects, what was a woman to do? Her book included sixteen interviews with practitioners of bio-identical hormone therapy. In 2006, she went on *The Oprah Winfrey Show*, and soon, in 2009, Oprah herself was describing how "menopause had caught her off guard" and that bio-identical hormones changed her life. Oprah had already waded into the menopause debate back in 2002, when she opened her show by looking into the camera and asking millions of women, "Are you in menopause . . . and don't know it?" This effectively started the national discussion of perimenopause. Her guest that episode was Christiane Northrup, a gynecologist and popular women's health advocate, and she said, "This is the PMS of the new millennium. It's something women have to pay attention to."[38] Now, four books later, Suzanne Somers is considered the guru of menopause, even though her approach is very similar to Robert Wilson's misogynistic take on menopause in his book, *Feminine Forever*.

Or is perimenopause another way to sell a product? As Dr. Anthony Scialli, professor of obstetrics and gynecology at the Georgetown University School of Medicine in Washington, D.C., stated, "Women's health has been phenomenally overmedicalized and commercialized."[39]

Yes, it has been—as we've seen—and this continues. With the menopause market peaking in 2003, drug companies worked furiously to replicate the success of Viagra, or Sildenafil, which is sold to treat erectile dysfunction. Erectile dysfunction is the inability to get or keep an erection. In 1998 Pfizer started selling Viagra, a vasodilator, to improve blood flow to the penis, as treatment for erectile dysfunction. While Viagra improves the mechanical part of erection, it does not help endocrine imbalance. Mechanics are only part of sexual stimulation. High levels of the hormone cortisol produced by the adrenal gland can interfere with sexual stimulation, for both men and women. Yet drug companies were immediately in search of the "female" version of Viagra. Sprout Pharmaceuticals had tried and failed to get its drug Flibanserin approved as an anti-depressant by FDA three times.[40] The company changed its marketing approach, and presented Flibanserin, now sold as Addyi, as treatment for hypoactive sexual desire disorder (HSDD) in women, a diagnosis that Ray Moynihan writing in the British Medical Journal in 2014 called obsolescent."[41]

With Viagra, Pfizer created the entirely new market of "sexual dysfunction," much the same way Wyeth did to sell Premarin and Prempro. In her documentary *Orgasm Inc.*, Liz Canner demonstrates how pharmaceutical companies jockeyed for FDA approval of a new drug to treat Female Sexual Dysfunction. This term was coined by drug companies and then promoted by paid "experts in the field" on morning talk shows, in newspapers, and in television news services. These "experts" reported that just under 50 percent of all women were sexually dysfunctional, meaning they had difficulty reaching orgasm. Forty-three percent soon became the accepted number among both doctors and journalists.

"Disease mongering" is another new term to come out of the study of the proliferation of invented illnesses. One executive, explaining her efforts to market new drugs, calls it "condition branding" or "multi-platform marketing." In the documentary *Orgasm Inc.*, the thirty-something executive smiles at the camera as the filmmaker asks how her company started developing a drug for Female Sexual Dysfunction (FSD). "We didn't even know what the disease was," she says. "In order for us to develop drugs, we need to better and more clearly define what the disease is."[42]

Just as our ability to procreate had to be kept under lock and key because of the property value of DNA, the loss of this procreative value, or menopause, came to be considered an illness. Only women, orcas, and pilot whales have the gift of menopause. Since the advent of agriculture society has viewed women and their reproductive value as an investment. When they could no longer produce offspring they lost value. Not for nothing did some cultures allow a man to have several wives. There is much literary, psychological, and sociological research into how women may have internalized the idea that once they are no longer reproductive they have outlived their usefulness. The media's desexualization of older women and the idealization of younger women reinforces this negative image of aging, but cannot explain away the physical symptoms women do experience.

It is hard to know if it started with symptoms, or possibly with a woman's fear of no longer being able to procreate. On the books, menopause seems to have been invented by men—specifically western men. Until recently, the term did not even exist in many other languages, but has since been imported into many Asian cultures. Research demonstrates that hot flashes and night sweats—the primary symptoms hormone therapy exists to treat—are rarely experienced by women in Asian countries. The rates of heart disease and osteoporosis—other symptoms the medical world insists hormone therapy is necessary to prevent—were consistently lower in such countries as Japan and China. This suggests that menopausal symptoms may also be culturally dependent and not the physiological boogeyman the West purports it to be. But menopausal symptoms *are* on the rise in Asia, as are diabetes and heart disease—two conditions also associated with women and aging.

Conclusion

The development of pharmaceuticals and the medicalization of menopause has been tied to commerce. Historically, the skewed approach to diagnosing women and treating them—first with surgery, then with hormones, then with psychoanalysis, then again with hormones and psycho-pharmaceuticals—has been perpetuated by the increase in the compartmentalization of medicine. The inventions of new branches of medicine—such as gynecology—further transformed symptoms not necessarily caused by a woman's reproductive system into newly named illnesses that required pharmaceutical treatment. With each new discovery in the endocrine system, a new drug was developed, which then required an illness for it to treat.

So what is a woman to do when she is in menopause? The word menopause is correct; it means menstruation stops, but this is not the reason for the symptoms she might be experiencing. Some writers have listed many more symptoms (as many as sixty-six on the UK doctor-sponsored medical information website Patient.info) than the seven dwarfs Suzanne Somers describes.[43] It isn't that there aren't any, but menopause is not the real reason for having them.

The symptoms women experience after menopause are indeed caused by hormones, but it's the imbalance of the endocrine system that wreaks havoc on our bodies, not the deficiency of one particular hormone, the estrogen produced in the ovaries. Endocrinology evolved from the concept that all factors for a woman's health were dictated by her reproductive organs and the hormones they produced. Before surgery was used to remove them, and before female sex hormones were isolated, some doctors treated women as a whole. They understood, without understanding how the endocrine system worked, that what a woman eats strongly influences her hormonal balance—the balance of the endocrine system. Unfortunately, doctors are no longer taught this; instead, they are taught to fight the female endocrine system with hormones derived from horse urine or synthetic hormones created in laboratories. They are forbidden to tell us that our lifestyles and what we eat are the primary factors in creating and maintaining endocrine balance. Research is a market, and healthcare has become a powerful industry that doctors and medical schools must serve to survive. Female humans evolved to have menopause as a way of living longer healthier lives. The meaning of the word has been distorted by medicine and by drug companies. It has been given a negative connotation and conjures up negative images. Women have been convinced that their bodies will let them down and that they will need drugs to enjoy what is the longest time of their lives. But it can be the best time of your life. Menopause is actually quite simple. So is how you can ensure you enjoy it.

CHAPTER TWO

Menopause Is Good

"It seems a pity to have a built-in rite of passage and to dodge it, evade it, and pretend nothing has changed. That is, to dodge and evade one's womanhood, to pretend one's like a man. Men, once initiated, never get the second chance. They never change again. That's their loss, not ours. Why borrow poverty?"

—Ursula K. Le Guin, "The Space Crone"

Menopause is good. This is because it gives us strength and allows us to slow aging. Halfway through her 2013 Margo Wilson Memorial Lecture, "Grandmothers and Human Evolution," at McMaster University in Ontario, Canada, Kristin Hawkes, a distinguished professor of anthropology, is about to explain how women differ from every other humanoid and all mammals except for orcas and pilot whales, when she says, "Here I am, a post-menopausal woman still." And she does a little jig.[1] "Here I am at my advanced age, more or less walking and chewing gum at the same time. If I was a chimpanzee I would have been dead decades ago."

She calls it the "fitness advantage," and explains that it is the evolution of menopause that gives humans the longevity that makes them so special and different. Hawkes and James O'Connell, a UCLA anthropologist, first published their research proposing the grandmother hypothesis in 1997. Their hypothesis states that as humans evolved in Africa over a period of two million years, the environment changed from rich forests, where newly weaned infants could collect food on their own, to dryer grasslands. "So moms had two choices," Hawkes explained in a *University of Utah News* interview. "They could either follow the retreating forests, where foods were available that weaned infants could collect, or continue to feed the kids after the kids are weaned."[2] This gave grandmothers, who were beyond their childbearing years, the important job of making food available, such as cracking open hard-shelled nuts or digging up tubers—work that small children did not have the physical strength to do. As has been seen in research into nineteenth- and twentieth-century Europeans and Canadians, in the Hazda (the Tanzanian people Hawkes and her colleagues studied) as well as in other African peoples, grandmothering increased their grandchildren's likelihood of survival.[3]

Women have always lived a very long time, Hawkes explains, and dispels the myth that that women did not live to be old, or "there didn't used to be any old people if you thought life expectancy was the measure of that."[4] The census data, such as that tracked by Oeppen and Vaupel and published in *Science* in 2002, is misleading.[5] Even though when Oeppen and Vaupel crunched the numbers for the Swedish of 1840 (Swedish women in 1840 had the longest life-expectancy) and arrived at a life expectancy of forty-four, an analysis compiled by Keyfitz and Flieger in 1968 shows that 34 percent of Swedish women in 1840 lived past age forty-five.[6] Women lived for decades after reaching menopause, and there is evidence that they lived longer when they were hunter-gatherers. It also shows that women who lived past fifteen had an 80 percent chance of living decades past fertility, and "most females did."[7]

Margaret Lock also addresses what she calls the myth that women rarely lived past middle age until the beginning of the twentieth century. "At the turn of the century a woman could expect to live to the age of forty-seven or eight"[8] Margaret Lock writes that in spite of the evidence that women have always survived several decades past menopause, "Nevertheless, the myth that women (men never appear in these arguments) dropped dead in their late forties is pervasive."[9] What is the reason for this? Life expectancy is measured by lumping together females of all ages. Medical statisticians use the reduced rate infant mortality and lowered mortality during childbirth to prove that increased life-expectancy is due to nutrition or improved public health care.[10] If a woman survived infancy and childbirth, she had a good chance of living past seventy. Medical texts reinforce the prejudiced notion that women living past their fertility is a new phenomenon and that medicine is playing catch-up to treat the symptoms that arrive with this new "unnatural" biology which is an "artifact" of our recent mastery of the environment.[11]

Kristin Hawkes describes how, in her studies of the Hazda tribe, she was surprised to find that "the old ladies were amazingly productive."[12] So much so that she was inspired to theorize that menopause drives the longevity of the human species and set to work proving the grandmother hypothesis in 1999 to explain the evolutionary quirk of menopause. Birds and bees don't do menopause.

According to medicine, a woman who lives past her childbearing years is an anomaly achieved by modern medicine. In addition to the grandmother hypothesis, there are several hypotheses for the origin of menopause. Another is the patriarch hypothesis from 2000, which describes the origin of menopause as allowing men to mate with younger women, supposedly resulting in increased longevity and increased status in society (for men); however, it does not explain why menopause evolved in the first place.[13] This theory is based on the assumption that men live longer than women—which, again, is false—taking us back to the original statistical error that a women lived until approximately forty-four. The assumption stems in part from the idea that men remain fertile in old age. Women stop bleeding, but men still have erections. Yet articles such as the one published on March 17, 2017, in the *World Economic Forum* continually ask the question "Why Do Women Live Longer Than Men?"[14] Studies are now changing the discourse surrounding the ever-productive man, a story certainly reinforced by the media (older men dumping their wives for younger, more "fertile" women to further the continuation of the human species). Sperm mobility decreases with age, and impotence increases. For this, Viagra was born. Studies show that human reproductive power actually starts to decline in the womb, but these studies do not get into the popular vernacular. Fun fact: a part of the male brain called the corpus callosum shrinks between the ages of twenty-four and seventy, while women's brains remain the same size.[15] The human being is biologically programmed to live for 110 years, and some scientists even say that humans have not come close to their full life-span potential. Menopause is evolutions's way of ensuring women live up to their life-span potential.

Surprised to find how the "old ladies were so critical economically,"[16] Kristin Hawkes used not only anthropological and evolutionary studies, but also endocrinology to make it clear that menopause is a major factor in the evolution of human longevity.

Lock writes that the arguments that women did not always live past menopause—that menopause causes both physical and mental decline—are disguising the ideological position that women exist only for the reproduction of the species. From the work of Kristin Hawkes and others, we see how important menopause is for longevity.

While the medical consensus is that women are programmed to keel over at forty-five, it is generally accepted that women live longer than men. The occasional magazine article tries to explain this, such as a 2008 *Time* article suggesting that women live longer because men burn out from an adolescent "testosterone storm," during which time they will engage in dangerous behavior such as "not wearing seat-belts."[17]

Women have always lived to a ripe old age, but certainly a higher percentage of them "got to be old people," as Kristin Hawkes demonstrates, in hunter-gatherer societies living on "wild food."[18] She says that in human history, agriculture happened "yesterday" (10,000 years ago), and therefore it is logical to study hunter-gatherer societies in order to determine why humans live so long.

Why are menopausal women seen (and why do they see themselves) as physically useless anomalies created by modern times, requiring medical care for the wide array of menopausal symptoms, such as osteoporosis? One study claims, "An unwelcome consequence of increased longevity, osteoporosis eventually develops in almost all untreated Caucasian women who reach their 80th year. The direct cost of osteoporotic fractures is estimated to be $7 billion to $10 billion each year in the United States alone, and the population of postmenopausal women is continually increasing."[19] So menopausal women aren't only miserable, they cost society money. Get them on hormone replacement therapy—or else to a nunnery.

Medicine uses various negative terms for menopause, including deficiency disease, endocrinopathy, ovarian failure, the menopausal syndrome, the climacteric syndrome, or simply regression. If menopause is something negative it will require something to make it better, and treatment from physicians who will the use ever-increasing pharmaceuticals for the ever-increasing number of symptoms.

Menopause treatment used to focus on the five to ten years after a woman actually stopped menstruating, but it has now become preventative, starting with treatment in perimenopause and extending far past menopause to postmenopause so as to prevent health care expenses due to brittle bones and heart disease.

What Is It, Really?

Menopause is the amazing evolution of human female longevity. Females of only three species of mammals go into menopause: orcas, pilot whales, and humans. Our closest primate relatives are reproductive until they die. So why did this amazing phenomenon evolve? Because it is so unusual, evolutionary anthropologists and biologists have done more research into menopause than modern medicine has. Menopause it is not a recent evolutionary change. This exceptional evolutionary selection took place because of the benefits of *not* having babies after a certain age. The age of menopause does not vary cross-culturally, ethnically, or historically. Japanese women go into menopause at about fifty. Aristotle in the fourth century BC wrote that it occurred at fifty years of age, as did Pliny, writing in the first century. Menopause has been around for a very long time.

Prenatal females have 7 million ovocytes. This number is reduced to two million at six months. At about five years old, it drops again to less than 500,000, followed by a much steadier decline until menopause.[20] By puberty, the time most associated with fertility, the number of ovocytes are further reduced to 400,000. When a woman ceases to menstruate, she only has about 1000 ovocytes left. Women are programmed to have a declining fertility. Artresia, a hormone withdrawal, causes the cell death of the follicles which produce the egg. Interestingly, Kristin Hawkes also discusses how girls getting their period later is another evolution that permits humans to live longer.

Our bodies are naturally programmed to stop menstruating, but we are also programmed to live a long time after the process has stopped. But us, orcas, and pilot whales? Why have the females of these three mammals evolved to live to grandmother our children's children? Because this way the grandchildren survive. While our reproductive system changes, everything else is supposed to thrive. Menopause just means no more babies.

As Hawkes wondered why "ancestral ovarian rates aged, but aging slowed in *other* [Hawkes's emphasis] physiological systems,"[21] Jared Diamond proposed in his book, *Why Sex is Fun*, that there must be an evolutionary reason for this.[22]

Since Darwin's laws of natural selection would seem to dictate that more time spent producing offspring benefits the species, menopause seemed like a strange strategy for Mother Nature to have chosen for the human female. Whereas our closest primate relatives age and decline physiologically, they remain reproductive until they die This is why the phenomenon of menopause so fascinates anthropologists and biologists. They consider all complex features of organisms to be the result of Darwinian natural selection, which means, to science, menopause is a fascinating adaptation. Why, they wondered, are human women born with a finite number of eggs? Why do their follicular reserves plummet prenatally when most other mammals, including other primates, have an unlimited amount in order to reproduce until death? Early humans, like women today, lived most of their lives in a post-reproductive state.

But being reproductive is hard work on many levels. Reproducing increases the need for energy and nutrients—both prenatally and after giving birth. And eating enough is difficult, because the fetus takes up space in the abdomen.[23] Organs remodel themselves to allow the fetus more space. Also, a woman's immune function is reduced during pregnancy to make up for the demands on her metabolism. Lactation also puts a huge demand on a woman's physiology.[24] Moms need help.

The premise of Kristin Hawkes's grandmother hypothesis is that grandmothers—menopausal women, who no longer had small children of their own—were there to help these moms. Menopause evolved precisely so more children in the family would survive.

We can also look to the other two known species in which menopause evolved. Orcas and pilot whales stop reproducing in their forties and can live into their nineties.

"Granny," the oldest known orca, is 103.[25] Studies using census data for killer whales of the Pacific Northwest, led by Ken Balcomb from the University of Exeter and Cambridge show that male orcas whose mothers live until a ripe old age are fourteen times more likely to live past thirty. Fertile killer whale females were three times as likely to die if their mothers died.[26] Evolution favors human female menopause, because more children are able to survive when their mothers give birth to fewer children. Men don't understand this, because they don't die in childbirth, and are less likely than women to exhaust themselves in caring for infants.

Evolution favors menopause. A grandmother can provide more hours of foraging than small children, new mothers, and teenagers. In the hunter-gatherer Hazda women Hawkes studied, foraging increased with experience and age. Even though they were older, the grandmothers' return on their foraging was higher than that of younger teenagers, and equal to that of reproductive women in their prime. Postmenopausal women could provide more food than younger women, and as this amount was far more than they could consume alone, their contribution was given to their close relatives.

Aside from foraging, grandmothers also babysat, as they often do today. In preliterate societies, postmenopausal women also served as libraries, contributing knowledge—about medicine, planting, and animals, for instance—that would benefit younger generations. The memories of an old woman could be very important to the survival of a tribe. This sort of contribution has also been seen in pilot whales—another species that experiences menopause. Granmother pilot whale "songs", help the whale pod find areas where the pods had foraged previously. Scientists found that postmenopausal orcas were "repositories of ecological knowledge."[27] Postmenopausal orcas make up a fifth of a whale pod (group) and more often lead the pod to food when it is scarce than younger females and males.[28]

Menopause is Mother Nature's crafty stratagem for carrying on her genes. Mitochondrial DNA, called maternal inheritance, is passed from mother to child, and occurs in humans and most multicellular organisms; however, the menopause gene is specific to just a few creatures, and in humans seems to be one of the most unusual of evolutionary strategies. There is a "Mitochondrial Eve," a woman from whom all living humans inherited their mitochondrial DNA,[29] and she naturally evolved to spend most of her life in menopause, so it makes no sense that it was supposed to be a drag.

CHAPTER THREE

Medicine for Menopause

"If any lady from thirty-five to fifty-five years of age is afflicted with dyspepsia, neuralgia, rheumatism, consumption or any other ailment, the doctor, not being able to cure her, pronounces it the menopause or 'change of life.'[1]

"Forget all the traditions and teachings upon this subject, and learn that nature creates no pathological conditions, and that if you live according to her laws you can by no possible means experience suffering."[2]

—Alice B. Stockham, *Tokology, a Book for Every Woman*

There is a section of the Mayo Clinic's website called "Diseases and Conditions, Menopause." In this section you will find their "Treatments and Drugs" page, on which the Mayo Clinic staff proclaims, "Menopause requires no medical treatment. Instead, treatments focus on relieving your signs and symptoms and preventing or managing chronic conditions that may occur with aging."[3]

Menopause is no longer the problem, then. Aging is. Still, it seems as though for women, aging is a particularly dangerous endeavor.

The Mayo Clinic defines menopause as the time when there has been no menstruation for twelve consecutive months and no other biological or physiological cause can be identified. The Mayo Clinic staff—like the writers for WebMD in the US, Patient.info in the UK, Sapere Salute in Italy, and Medisite in France—maintain that, excepting surgical menopause, menopause is a natural phase in a woman's life. Yet, as stated on the Mayo Clinic page, "The physical symptoms, such as hot flashes, and emotional symptoms of menopause may disrupt your sleep, lower your energy or—for some women—trigger anxiety or feelings of sadness and loss. Don't hesitate to seek treatment for symptoms that bother you. Many effective treatments are available, from lifestyle adjustments to hormone therapy."[4] Though I am sure the Mayo Clinic does indeed suggest lifestyle adjustments, medicine is still their business.

The common symptoms, both physical and emotional, listed on all of these sites and supposedly requiring medical treatment, include:

Irregular periods

Vaginal dryness

Hot flashes

Night sweats

Sleep problems

Mood changes

Weight gain and slowed metabolism

Thinning hair and dry skin

Loss of breast fullness

The UK's Patient.info helpfully lists sixty-six symptoms associated with menopause. And if experience has taught us anything about the medical industry, more symptoms will be added to that list as researchers discover ever more receptor sites activated by estrogen. Historically, medical professionals have defined menopause as a deficiency disease. The medical industry has consistently propagated the idea that menopause, as a period of non-productivity, is a negative event that requires treatment, through drugs or surgery, as if living into middle age is an accident of nature. To researchers, doctors, and pharmaceutical companies whose working hypothesis is that a reduction means a deficiency, the discovery of more receptor sites would signify that more places in a woman's body would suffer from the reduced production of estrogen.

Estrogen hormones do have significant effects on a woman's body, but estradiol (E2), is the only one whose production is reduced significantly in menopause. It is however still synthesized from estrone. A small amount of Estradiol is synthesized in the ovaries, where it is then primarily involved in maintaining the lining of the uterus and inducing the release of luteinizing hormone. Here estradiol triggers ovulation, and ovulation only. But estradiol is still synthesized from estrone, the hormone more prevalent after menopause. There are many estrogen receptors in the female body. Researchers keep finding more. Each time a new place where estrogen would seem to bind to promote a physiological function in our bodies—such as the estrogen receptors found in brain tissue— an alarm is raised, and drug company researchers hypothesize that this function will deteriorate without enough estrogen. But all those estrogen receptors they keep finding bind not only to the estradiol produced in the ovaries. If 75 percent of estrogen(s) are synthesized in peripheral tissue prior to menopause, rising to 80 percent after menopause, the math clearly states that ovarian production only makes up for 5 percent. The female body did not use ovarian estradiol to bind to estrogen receptors previously, and it does not need it to bind to them after menopause.

When the University of Rochester Medical Center, a major medical research institution, writes on its online health encyclopedia, "The woman's ovaries make most estrogen hormones, although the adrenal glands and fat cells also make small amounts of the hormones," they omit the fact that they specifically mean estradiol and not estrogen.

Medical literature claims all estrogenic effects decline significantly with the reduction of estradiol. Medicine interprets this to mean the sites where estrogen receptors are found will not be stimulated, and that the tissues, organs, and physiological systems that function by binding to estrogen will go into withdrawal. Not only that, but since ovarian production declines in a woman's thirties, the literature attests that these symptoms "may" appear as early as age thirty-five. This was why "perimenopause" was invented. As Dr. Tony Scialli, professor of obstetrics and gynecology at Georgetown University, put it in 2003, "The term perimenopause became popular among health care providers and the media only a few years ago. Creating a medical term has invited medical researchers to take ownership of the condition and thereby to study it. Unfortunately, such studies require that criteria be invented for defining a condition, and particular creativity is involved when the condition itself is invented."[5]

It would seem that simply being a woman inherently requires medication. Medicine has always medicalized menopause, and the isolation of the estrogen hormone in 1928 made this much easier to do. Gynecology textbooks describe menopause as a change women "dread" and that they "fear the onset of uncomfortable physical side effects and loss of their youth."[6] So what does this decline in ovarian estrogen production really mean for the female body?

The primary change to reproductive function is the decline in ovarian follicle regeneration. Follicles decrease in number and then no longer produce eggs. This is a mechanical alteration, functioning primarily to end a woman's ability to procreate. The three different estrogen hormones: estrone (E1), estradiol (E2), and estriol (E3) all originate from androgens, specifically testosterone and androstenedione, which is synthesized by the enzyme aromatase in the adrenals.[7] The difficulty arises from the fact that estrogen was discovered some years before adrenal hormones. Edward C. Kendall and his colleagues worked for twenty years to isolate many hormones produced in the adrenal glands, and there may still be more even as-yet-undiscovered hormones produced in these glands. Remember, endocrinology is a new science. Estrogen was discovered in 1929. Both Edward A. Doisy and Adolf Butenandt isolated it in the same year. Pharmaceutical companies funded their research from the beginning with a clear intent to synthesize and sell it. With every new hormone discovered, it becomes more and more clear that the endocrine system and how it relates to different processes in the body is far more complicated than a simple cause-and-effect reaction.

Estradiol production decreases in the ovaries, but adrenal, liver, muscle, breast, and fat tissue are already involved in a large part of estradiol hormone synthesis throughout a woman's whole life. All three estrogens start off as cholesterol. Estradiol is the last estrogen hormone synthesized. When the ovaries reduce production, the adrenals producing 85 percent of androstenedione, will (with properly functioning adrenals and a diet with sufficient cholesterol, or fat) take over most of the estrogen synthesis.[8] Since a woman's body specifically evolved to remain fertile for only a limited period of time, estradiol production must no longer be necessary for a woman's well-being after menopause.

Cholesterol, which is made in the liver, serves as the source for steroids from which the three major estrogens (estrone, estradiol, and estriol) are synthesized. Vital to this process is the enzyme aromatase, which is responsible for converting androgens into estrogens. The aromatase enzyme can be found in many tissues, including adipose, blood, and bone tissue. However, high cortisol and insulin levels—often caused by a high-carbohydrate diet—and estrogen dominance, or estrogen resistance, caused by xenoestrogens, can disrupt this conversion. In that case, the adrenals will not be able to produce estrone (E1). Researchers, pharmaceutical companies, and doctors, in that order (or perhaps I should rephrase it as researchers researching for pharmaceutical companies), only focus on estradiol (E2)—the production of which does indeed decline in the ovaries with menopause. Though, as we have seen earlier, E2 actually starts to decline in the womb, but that ruins their argument.

Estrogens spread readily across cell membranes. As they enter diverse kinds of cells, they must bind to and activate estrogen receptors. It is the binding of estrogens to many cells that makes its production important for a woman's health and vitality. Medical research primarily focuses on the cause and effect of reduced production of estrogen by the ovaries, and consequently, the theoretical reduction of estrogens binding to different cells. This completely ignores the built-in safety mechanism of the adrenals in the female endocrine system, i.e.: the production of non-ovarian sources of estrogen. These non-ovarian sources of estrogen prevent menopausal symptoms and are what should make menopause a vital and productive time in a woman's life. Since the discovery of reproductive hormones at the turn of the century, physicians have been trained more and more to believe that women suffer from severe symptoms that require clinical attention. Plus, the damaging images used in the first advertisements for hormone replacement drugs have furthered this negative perception of menopause. Medications were initially approved to treat only hot flashes, a side effect suffered by a minority of women—many of whom had been subjected to surgical menopause, many of them victims of the surgical menopause craze, as well as those rare cases of women born without ovaries. Charles Dodds, the inventor of diethylstilbestrol—the first non-steroidal estrogen—never intended it to be used on healthy women.

Today, menopause is marketed as a life-threatening disease that endangers most women through a variety of illnesses, including breast cancer and heart disease. A Medscape slideshow includes images showing the disintegration of bone tissue, along with the following statement: "Alteration of hormone profiles during and after the onset of menopause can also exert multiple effects on various organ systems. For example, low estrogen levels can lead to atrophy of hormone-dependent tissue areas (eg, vagina and external genitalia). Hormonal changes can also result in marked redistribution of fat and thickening of facial hair. Perhaps the most medically concerning process caused by menopausal hormone fluctuations is the increased rate of bone mineral density (BMD) loss, particularly during the 3 years surrounding the final menstrual period."[9] Disease mongering? I think so.

While the symptoms associated with menopause have increased in the last fifty years, as has their gravity, the word "treatment" has all but disappeared from English-language medical literature since the July 2002 halt of the Women's Health Initiative's trial of estrogen plus progestin therapy. A frightening number of trial participants suffered the diseases the hormone therapy was intended to prevent. In the 1970s, the women's health movement influenced the way in which pharmaceutical companies attempted to frame the word "menopause." Menopause is no longer a disease, but a condition with symptoms that require "management." Beginning in 1970, the phrase "treating menopause" rose dramatically in English publications, peaking in 2000, and then dropping significantly in 2005, whereas the words "managing menopause" are only seen in English-language publications after the year 2000, with their use continually increasing (according to the Google Ngram Viewer, which plots the usage of words and phrases in publications).

So how is management accomplished? "Management" means pharmaceuticals, such as hormone replacement therapy, antidepressants, anti-seizure medications, and vaginal lubricants as medical treatment.

Hormone Therapy

Emminem, made from the urine of pregnant women, went on the market in 1933. It was prescribed for gonorrheal vaginitis, atrophic vaginitis, and hot flashes. Diethylstilbestrol (DES) was approved by the FDA in 1941 and marketed as a far more powerful estrogen. In 1942, the FDA approved the sale of Ayerst's Premarin—made from the urine of pregnant horses and even more powerful than DES—as a treatment for hot flashes. Since that time, synthetic hormones have become synonymous with treating not only the symptoms associated with menopause but the symptoms of aging in general. Yet estrogen therapy is actually estrone therapy. The urine from pregnant mares (or from pregnant women) does not provide estradiol—the deficiency of which hormone therapy is sold to treat—and so it does not replace the body's supposed lack of estradiol. Estrone, or E1, is produced at the same low level in pregnancy as in menopause. Therefore, hormone therapy in the form of conjugated estrogens is simply taking what women's bodies produce naturally, but from an outside source, and lots more of it. The larger quantities, or the super potency of the conjugated estrogens, has always been what was most dangerous about them. Medicine—as represented by doctors, researchers, and drug manufacturers—took the simplified idea that if something is good, a lot of it must be better, and thereby created an industry.

The history of conjugated estrogens—the bestselling hormone therapy—has had its ups and down. Conjugated estrogens have been marketed as the fountain of youth for women, even though the health risks of the use of exogenous hormones had been known from the time of their development. These findings were kept to medical journals and research papers, which were written and read by men, until the 1960s and '70s, when the feminist movement in the United States inspired women to inform themselves about their health. Only then did the dangers of hormone replacement therapy reach the public. Finally, women's health groups were able to stand up to the powerful drug lobbies that had historically used their influence to gain government approval for drugs marketed to women. The marketing of hormone therapy has always been brilliant and has often influenced—if not mirrored—how women see themselves. After the 1970s, many women no longer identified with the drug companies' image of the withered and useless crone. And even though the emancipated woman took control of her own health, still those same companies were able to turn this against her.

Manufacturers initially advertised to women who went into menopause. Women in their fifties were told that they could regain their spark by taking hormones to replace the ones they had lost to menopause. This approach changed in 1964, when Ayerst ran its first advertisement promoting Premarin as a long-term hormone replacement therapy.[10] Still, the national discourse about the powers of information manufacturers and doctors had over patients was changing.

The Kefauver-Harris Bill requiring drug manufacturers to provide proof of their drug's effectiveness as well as its safety, passed in 1962 amending the Federal Food, Drug, and Cosmetic Act in the aftermath of the thalidomide tragedy. Thalidomide was a German-made sedative prescribed to women in Europe and Australia during pregnancy; due to the side effects, thousands of babies were born with missing or malformed limbs. My mother lived in New York when she was pregnant with me, but in 1965 we moved to Germany. I went to kindergarten with several of these children, and I remember how impressed I was by a little boy who could draw much better than I could, using only his feet. Thalidomide was never approved by the US FDA; Dr. Frances O. Kelsey, head of the agency's new Office of Scientific Investigations and personally appointed by President Kennedy, had been troubled by some data on thalidomide. While following up on the research submitted by the William S. Merrell Company, Kelsey discovered that studies had been omitted from Merrell's approval application. Consequently, Kelsey delayed approval until she could study the research herself. In the months that followed, while representatives from the manufacturer inundated Kelsey's superiors with complaints about the delay, reports of horrific birth defects began to surface in the countries where the drug had been legalized. Kelsey's refusal to cave to industry pressure saved thousands of children.[11]

"Her exceptional judgment in evaluating a new drug for safety for human use has prevented a major tragedy of birth deformities in the United States," President John F.

Kennedy said of Frances O. Kelsey during a White House ceremony in her honor.[12]

Over the next few years, the power of the FDA increased, and the public—especially women—wanted more information about the drugs they were being prescribed. Prior to the Kefauver-Harris amendment, women simply followed their doctors' instructions and the suggestions of the advertising directed at them. The facts about a drug's efficacy and possible health risks were not available to consumers, as manufacturers did not have to put warning labels on packages or include informational inserts. It wasn't until 1979 that the FDA ruled that manufacturers would be compelled to include in the packaging a pamphlet outlining the health risks for estrogen therapy. Estrogen therapy became one of only four drugs required by the FDA to contain warnings. The other three were contraceptives, progestin, and an asthma inhaler.[13] No other drugs were required to carry warning labels at the time.

With the passage of the Kefauver-Harris amendment, drug companies now had to demonstrate not only the efficacy of their prescription drugs, but also their safety. Additionally, the FDA could now control medical advertising. At the Joint Hearings before the Subcommittee on Health in 1976, chaired by Senator Edward Kennedy, Kennedy made it clear that what he'd heard during the committee had convinced him that the medical and pharmaceutical industry was a danger to the American public. He described an advertisement for Premarin in *Medical World News,* the tagline of which was: "While you are calming her down with a tranquilizer, treat what may be her real problem with Premarin."[14] At the senate subcommittee, eleven FDA employees testified that they had been harassed by the drug industry and that industry pressure influenced the investigations of the research the drug companies submitted.[15]

In 1970, the FDA wrote the first label insert for oral contraceptives; using language that patients could easily understand, they outlined the health risks and twenty-five side effects to be on the lookout for. Unfortunately, the FDA ultimately bowed to pressure from both manufacturers and doctors, who complained that the informational insert would interfere with the doctor–patient relationship.[16] At the senate hearings, some doctors complained that women would not even be able understand the information provided and that the doctors' time would be wasted assuaging their patients' fears inspired by the insert.

In 1975, the *New England Journal of Medicine* published two articles that demonstrated a four- to fourteen-times increased risk of endometrial cancer with postmenopausal use of conjugated hormone therapy. After meeting with the FDA's Advisory Committee on Obstetrics and Gynecology in 1976 to discuss the studies, Ayerst sent doctors a letter reassuring them that Premarin was safe to prescribe, minimizing the risk of uterine and endometrial cancer with prolonged use of estrogen therapy. Furious, *FDA Drug Bulletin* published a statement condemning the irresponsible "Dear Doctor" letter. The battle between the FDA and the medical industry continued with consumer groups demanding more information from drug companies. The National Women's Health Network argued, "Citizens need to know about these risks and benefits in order to make an informed decision."[17] Drug labeling soon became a feminist issue.[18]

An informational insert, abridged from six pages down to one hundred words, was finally included in birth control packages starting in 1979. However, when estrogen prescriptions were filled by pharmacists, the information about hormone therapy as treatment for menopause was handed out as a separate pamphlet at the time the prescription was filled. According to FDA researchers working as undercover agents, only 39 percent of US pharmacists gave out the pamphlet. Still, Premarin sales dropped from twenty-eight million in 1975 to fourteen million in 1980, even though less than half of the prescriptions filled included the risk information.

Certainly the extended media coverage in the late 1970s about the risks of endometrial cancer caused more women to change their mind about estrogen therapy. Many women wrote to the senate subcommittee complaining that they had been given Premarin for decades: "I've gotten to the point where my faith in doctors and pills is at an all time low ebb. So please, print the warnings already—my money doesn't grow on trees."[19] Another wrote saying, "I took Premarin for ten years and found that it was the reason for ten years of headaches which sent me to the hospital many times. I finally got tired of Premarin and found to my surprise that I no longer had headaches. It cost me a fortune in medical bills which labeling could have prevented. Why did I take it in the first place??? Because some doctor probably had stock in American Home Products?"[20] Premarin's days as the top-selling drug in the United States seemed to be over.

Common side effects of conjugated estrogen therapy—none of which were listed until 1979—include:

Stomach upset or cramps

Nausea

Vomiting

Bloating

Breast tenderness or swelling

Headache

Weight or appetite changes

Freckles or darkening of facial skin

Increased hair growth

Loss of scalp hair

Problems with contact lenses

Vaginal itching or discharge

Changes in your menstrual periods

Decreased sex drive

Nervousness

Dizziness

Feeling tired

Mental/mood changes (such as depression and memory loss)

Breast lumps

Unusual vaginal bleeding (such as spotting, breakthrough bleeding, prolonged or recurrent bleeding)

Increased/ new vaginal irritation/itching/odor/discharge

Severe stomach or abdominal pain

Persistent nausea or vomiting

Yellowing eyes or skin

Dark urine

Swelling of hands/ankles/feet

Increased thirst

Frequent urination

Drug companies, always brilliant at reshaping the discourse, were able to steer the discussion from the use of estrogen as treatment for menopause to the *prevention* of menopause. Osteoporosis studies were conducted with estrogen, which seemingly proved that estrogen therapy improved bone density in women in their twenties and thirties. This new possibility of preventing menopause through estrogen influenced the National Institute of Health to convene the Consensus Development Conference in 1984; this was chaired by a doctor who later became a paid advisor to companies that manufactured pharmaceuticals and machinery that measured bone density. What was left out of the discussion was that the research had not been done on healthy menopausal women but on women who'd undergone oophorectomies in their twenties and thirties. Sales for Premarin, which had slumped dramatically over a five-year period, once again skyrocketed.

In 1992, manufacturers discovered they could remove the implication that estrogen increased a woman's risk of cancer by including in their products synthetic progesterone, or progestin, to mimic the natural rise and fall of hormones in a woman's cycle. This therapy was approved in Europe several years before it was approved in the US, because manufacturers were able to set up clinical trials much more easily in Europe than in the US. "Estrogen therapy" became "hormone therapy." As this was simply a combination of two synthetically combined hormones that had already been approved separately, the FDA approved Prempro in 1994. Prempro was put on the market without a randomized clinical trial in the US.

After the debacle of Women's Health Initiative in 2002, it was not the first time the use of combined estrogen and progesterone therapy was maligned by both doctors and women. But the lucrative practice of rebranding and off-label marketing engaged in first by Ayerst, then Wyeth-Ayerst, and now Pfizer, seems to ensure that hormone replacement therapy remains the "gold standard" treatment for menopause. "Off-label" means the use of pharmaceutical drugs for the treatment of symptoms with no proof of efficacy or safety from the FDA. It only takes a few papers—produced by researchers working in university labs funded by pharmaceutical companies, and hawked by lobbyists—to convince doctors, and even nations, that they should tell women that hormone replacement therapy will be of benefit to them. Furthermore, the practice of approving drugs in Europe and then using that same research to gain approval in the United States has been common since the 1960s. Remember, it took the formidable Frances O. Kelsey to spot the omissions in the research Merrell presented to approve thalidomide as a sedative for morning sickness. Alexander M. Schmidt, who served as commissioner of the FDA during the Nixon and Ford presidency, resented that the drug industry accused his agency of taking too long to approve new drugs.[21]

He said, "At that time, it depended in part on where the pre-clinical work was done, where the clinical studies were done, what data—FDA was then not accepting foreign data. A lot of drug companies were starting their drugs out in Europe because it was easier to do clinical studies there than in the U.S., and they were registering drugs first in other countries before they even submitted an NDA in the U.S."[22] Alexander Schmidt said that FDA labeling also served to protect the drug industry from litigation.

In 1997, Wyeth-Ayerst (before it was acquired by Pfizer, thereby becoming the largest pharmaceutical behemoth in the world) teamed up with the American Heart Association to launch a new initiative focused on women and heart disease. "Take Wellness To Heart would be a 'multi-faceted campaign,'" to quote Wyeth-Ayerst's own press release, "which will raise awareness that heart disease is the number one cause of death of women—killing more than 500,000 women annually."[23] The campaign targeted menopausal and postmenopausal women and coincided with a Wyeth-Ayerst-funded Heart and Estrogen-Progestin Replacement Study (which made the cute acronym HERS), to examine if hormone therapy would reduce the frequency of new cardiovascular disease.

It is because of these claims, and because of their lack of warnings, that in 2014 Pfizer was ordered to pay $330 billion in lawsuits brought by women who were seeking protection from heart disease and osteoporosis, and instead got breast-, ovarian-, and gallbladder cancer, lupus, Non-

Hodgkin's lymphoma, strokes, scleroderma, venous thrombosis, pulmonary embolism, and asthma.[24] In 2003, the FDA slapped black label box warnings—the strictest label the FDA can put on a drug when there is evidence of an association of a serious health risk—on all HRT products.

In spite of this, the medical industry still claims that synthetic hormones remain the best treatment for menopause. A recent *National Menopause Society* article was titled "The Experts Do Agree About Hormone Therapy."[25] These experts were the North American Menopause Association, which begat the International Menopause Association—both founded by Dr. Wolf Utian, who received payments from Wyeth-Pfizer. The International Menopause Society publishes a medical journal called *Climacteric,* which they claim "has become a leader in publishing peer-reviewed research on the menopause."[26]

Since 2002—and the well-publicized health risks associated with hormone therapy—Pfizer has been able to pivot its marketing and research by creating bazedoxifene. Bazedoxifene was first approved in European Medicines Agency in 2009 and marketed by itself with the brand name Conbriza to treat osteoporosis in menopausal women. In their section about how to use Conbriza, EMA's website adds that vitamin D and calcium supplements should be taken with Conbriza as research proves that vitamin D and mineral deficiencies are more to blame for bone demineralization than aging.[27] Bazedoxifene is marketed as a selective estrogen receptor modulator (SERM), meaning that it binds to only certain estrogen receptors and not to others. The hypothesis is that bazedoxifene will bind to those receptors that will improve some symptoms associated with menopause, thereby improving hot flashes and bone density, but "may" not (according to researchers whose studies Pfizer included in its approval application) increase cell growth in the uterus or in breast tissue.[28]

A study published in *Therapeutics and Clinical Risk Management concluding the positive effects of bazedoxifene* in

2008 was written by researchers who reference their own past studies, as well as other studies conducted by researchers working at universities whose research departments are funded by Pfizer. For instance one of the main European researchers for bazedoxifene is Doris Gruber of the Obstetrics and Gynecology Department for the University of Vienna, one of Wyeth Europe's (a Pfizer subsidiary) main research labs. In a 2011 interview, Pfizer's Anthony Coyle—who was heading up an aggressive program to increase drug-development-ready research from universities in Europe, Asia, and the United States—said the conglomerate wants to speed up the process of defining the mechanism of a drug's action at the same time as it is developing the appropriate drug that will target the process in the body, and determine the right patient population to target it to. In 2011, Pfizer's goal was to "bring dozens of differentiated biologics against new targets into the clinical pipeline," and this means giving a lot of money to academia.[29] Coyle also said that by speeding up the process, Pfizer will be able to bypass the step of animal testing, which will bring drugs to human clinical trials much faster, and will thus speed up the approval process. Pfizer wants this deeper collaboration with university research teams to get drugs through testing in five years. This will mean there will be less time for side effects and health risks to become apparent. Short-term profits seem to bring in more revenue than what the company loses in paying damages.

Interestingly, the FDA still has not approved bazedoxifene for use in the US by itself. Wyeth tried to get it approved in 2008, calling it Viviant. In 2009, Pfizer bought Wyeth and inherited the Wyeth line of hormone therapy drugs. In 2010, Viviant was approved for use in Japan, but not in America. So what did Pfizer do? It combined bazedoxifene with conjugated estrogen, and in 2013, Duavee received FDA approval—despite the predictions of market analysts, given the bad press surrounding hormone therapy after 2001.[30] Duavee was approved to treat vasomotor symptoms and postmenopausal osteoporosis. A lot has changed in the FDA's approval process since Alexander

Schmidt was commissioner during the 1970s. The FDA now more readily accepts clinical trials conducted in foreign countries. Drug companies are globally owned, so drug companies which have invested in foreign research can submit that research to the FDA for approval.

Common side effects of Duavee:

Muscle spasms

Dizziness

Nausea

Diarrhea

Dyspepsia

Abdominal pain

Neck pain

Throat pain

Vaginal Estrogen

Ancient medicine focused on the body as a closed-energy system—in other words, all organs are in competition for nourishing and oxygenating blood. In Galen's time, women were considered "wet" and "damp" because they menstruated; wetness was associated with fertility. In the nineteenth century, when surgeons began removing women's reproductive organs, it was assumed that women would "dry up." Now that women had been ousted from the midwife profession and were not yet allowed in medical schools, male surgeons exaggerated the roles of the uterus and ovaries and claimed they were competing with the rest of the body for a limited quantity of blood.

In 1937, Robert M. Lewis wrote that in "menopause or castration the vaginal mucosa reverts to the thin, ill developed structure of childhood."[31] The cause, according to Lewis, was a reduction in acidity, which led to infection and thus produced burning, itching, and pain during intercourse. Lewis began experimenting with estrogen in 1933, when he injected the vaginal tissue of female children with an estrogen substance to find out if "it was possible to change the thin vaginal mucosa of the child to that resembling the thick epidermis-like structure of the adult."[32] The "large amounts" of the estrogenic substance Lewis used was amniotin, provided by E. R. Squibb, and Lewis conducted his experiments on patients at Bellevue Pediatric Hospital, New York's first psychiatric hospital, infamous for its experimentation on children.[33] Lewis defined "senile vaginitis," as the inflammation of vaginal mucosa in older women due to a deficiency in estrogen. Lewis did mention that the treatment was "possibly injurious, although there is no conclusive evidence of harmful results following such treatment."[34]

K. J. Karnaky also used amniotin, or stilbestrol, in his research on younger women, often girls, suffering from gonorrhea.[35] After Charles Dodds published the formula for dieythylstilbestrol in 1938, Karnaky prescribed it to thousands of pregnant women to prevent uterine bleeding—even though Dodds sent him a report stating that DES would actually *cause* uterine bleeding.[36] The term senile vaginitis was coined in the late 1930s. In 1963, Henry Falk, MD, described it as a misnomer in the *Journal of the American Geriatrics Society*, because it related not to infection, but to the atrophy of vaginal tissue. Falk considered vaginal atrophy to be one of the many "vaginal disorders caused primarily by lowered estrogen production," the more cases of which are due to the "40% increase in the aging female population."[37]

Withering and drying up are supposed to be the consequences of aging, while young and pulpy embodied fertility. Research into the medical applications of estrogen was driven by male preconceptions about femininity. It was this self-fulfilling prophecy that made menopause into an illness. Atrophic vaginitis was a side effect experienced by women who had undergone hysterectomies, and early uses of vaginal estrogens were used to treat the sudden endocrine imbalance. Its use as a treatment for menopause was an early off-label application. One of the medicines for atrophic vaginitis was Schering's Dienestrol cream, introduced in the US in 1947; Dienestrol cream was a close analog of DES, which caused breast cancer in women exposed to it in utero and which is 200 to 400 percent more potent than the estradiol the body produces.[38]

As of 2001, WebMD was still suggesting Ortho Dienestrol Cream to treat "Vaginal Inflammation due to Loss of Hormone Stimulation, Painful Sexual Intercourse due to Menopause, Wasting of Tissues of the Vulva." In 2005, Ortho Dienestrol Cream was discontinued in the US. One of the side effects for Vagifem—an estrogen tablet made by Novo Nordisk, the most used widely used estrogen replacement drug in Europe and the US—is vaginal itching, which is one of the symptoms Vagifem is supposed to treat!

Common side effects of Vagifem:

Nausea

Stomach cramps

Vomiting

Bloating

Diarrhea

Breast swelling or tenderness

Nipple discharge

Vaginal itching or discharge

Swelling of ankles or feet

Headache (including migraines)

Changes in weight

Dizziness

Cold symptoms

Changes in skin color

Increased facial hair

Thinning scalp hair

Depression

WebMD, which lists these symptoms on the WedMD owned and operated site RxList, states that it is vital to "tell your doctor if you have serious side effects of Vagifem including: mental/mood changes (such as depression, memory loss), breast lumps."[39] RxList's "Vagifem" page offers an immediate warning, stating that Vagifem is an estrogen therapy and therefore increases the risk of endometrial cancer, cardiovascular disorders, breast cancer, and dementia. Good to know.

In 2007, Medscape (also owned by WebMD), the online resource for doctors and health professionals, published an article titled "Vaginal Atrophy: The 21st Century Health Issue Affecting Quality of Life: Special Populations," written by Michael L. Krychman, MD. The article proclaimed that vaginal dryness and atrophy is a silent epidemic affecting 50 to 60 percent of postmenopausal women, who have chosen to suffer in silence due to embarrassment and cultural taboos. "Younger" women and perimenopausal women may also experience periodic vaginal dryness and associated problems."[40]

The North American Menopause Society recommends the use of low-dose estrogen as the first line of treatment. Starting on the second page of the Medscape article itself, after the part about the best treatment being a low-dose estrogen, a sentence on the bottom of the page states that the article's entirety was "Supported by an independent educational grant from Novo Nordisk." Novo Nordisk, as we know, is the Danish multinational pharmaceutical company that manufactures Vagifem.

Even though conjugated estrogens have been on the market for seventy years, Pfizer's conjugated estrogen products are extremely expensive. In an attempt to explain the reason for this, the People's Pharmacy wrote in a 2016 online article that the complexity of its biotechnology has made it difficult for the FDA to approve a generic form of the drug. The uniqueness and complexity of this biological medicine has made it hard for the FDA to approve any generic substitutes.[41] Years ago, a three-month supply of Premarin cost $7. In the United States today, a month's supply costs $140. As a result, many Americans try to buy Premarin in Canada. In 2016, a *New York Times* article described how a woman who had been prescribed Vagifem resorted to ordering 90 tablets from a Canadian pharmacy; these were then impounded at the Los Angeles International Airport for being an illegal drug.[42] The cost for a year's supply of Vagifem in the US? $1000. In Canada? $100. In European countries, hormone therapy is covered by national health insurance, but governments must still pay full price for the drugs. Either way, the cost is astronomical, both monetarily and physically.

Antidepressants/SRRI Drugs

In 1686, fourteen "witches" were executed in Salem, Massachusetts—thirteen of them menopausal women. In Victorian England, menopausal women were considered mentally deranged, suffering from incurable dementia. Dr. Lawson Tait, a London gynecologist, was criticized for casually removing women's ovaries and tubes to bring on menopause for the relief of "neuroses, menstrual, psychic or physical symptoms"[43]; he was also the origin of Tait's Law, which went: "When in doubt, open the belly to find out!"[44] In his opinion, relief could be achieved by the use of "an occasional purgative" and "removal from home at frequent intervals," which meant being sent to a psychiatric institution.[45] Hundreds of Victorian women died under the knife during and following complications from the surgeries that became a commonplace cure for the female "nervous" condition. Isaac Baker Brown, a gynecologist, went further than the accepted removal of the uterus and the ovaries. He performed the clitoridectomy on his patients, even writing a book titled *The Curability of Certain Forms of Insanity, Epilepsy, Catalepsy, and Hysteria in Females* in 1866.[46] Brown was denounced by his colleagues, not because of the barbarity of the surgery, but because his peers were jealous of his success.[47]

But sedatives soon became the "gold standard" to treat the supposed emotional disturbances that plagued women at this time. Of course, once estrogen was discovered, sedatives took a backseat to hormone therapy's promise of a cure-all for menopause—aside from psychotherapy's short stint as the chosen treatment for menopausal depression and mood swings. Equine and synthetic estrogens were already the bestselling drugs for many pharmaceutical companies because of their brilliant marketing, but in the 1950s some drug companies selling sedatives tried to compete with hormone therapy Since a woman's "nervous effects" hurt not only her but the whole family (as illustrated by a Merrell advertisement featuring a woman berating her husband, while their teenage daughter consoles him), manufacturers of sedatives battled it out in magazines. With taglines such as "Now she can cope," for the barbiturate Butisol (directed at husbands) and "In the menopause . . . transition without tears . . . ." for Milprem (directed at women), drug companies made sure the whole family was involved. A Premarin advertisement directed at doctors declared, "Doctors too like Premarin."

One advertisement for a sedative declared, "The majority of menopausal women require no endocrine treatment at all."[48] Some doctors agreed. In the 1950s, there were still some doctors who preferred the three-tier approach of first counseling, then sedatives, and only then, if that didn't work, hormone therapy. But, in 1958, Elwood Jensen discovered the estrogen receptor. This made it clear that estrogen hormones were involved in more than reproduction and that estrogen stimulated a variety of tissues and physiological processes. But rather than take a closer look at how other parts of the endocrine system affected women's health, manufacturers and researchers instead invested time and money into finding new clinical applications for estrogen therapy.[49]

Then in 2002 all the theories about the benefits of hormone therapy for healthy women, women who were simply aging, that had remained unimpeachable since its birth, came crashing down. The claims had gotten bolder and bolder. In the nineties, Wyeth-Ayerst went beyond their initial claims that hormone therapy would stop hot flashes and prevent osteoporosis, saying that it would also reduce the incidence of heart attack and ischemia in women. In 2002, the Women's Health Initiative's clinical trials—intended to finally get to the bottom of all the unsubstantiated claims about the hormones—were halted. As a result many women were afraid to take hormones and many doctors were afraid to prescribe them. Pharmaceutical companies were consolidating into only a few corporations: Wyeth swallowed Ayerst, Pfizer swallowed Wyeth, etc. Big Pharma was born. Today most pharmaceuticals are made by only a handful of global companies. After the WHI report, even more money was spent on research in finding benefits for hormone therapy to fill in the immediate gap due to the drop in sales.

It gets especially confusing, because all of these medications supposedly treat more than one symptom. WebMD states that some antidepressants not only improve mood, but also "may" reduce hot flashes. Premarin vaginal cream, prescribed to treat vaginal atrophy and vaginal dryness, also helps hot flashes. Duavive, which is the Italian name for Duavee, advertises that it improves vaginal dryness.[50] This is described as symptom management for women who, "for health reasons," cannot take estrogen. Women who have had hysterectomies are advised that they can take estrogen, since the organ in which it has been proven to cause cancer is gone. Women who still have at least one ovary are advised that they can take the combined therapy of estrogen and progestin, because progestin will nullify the risk of cancer. It doesn't make sense. It made even less sense when, according to the WHI report, women taking the combined therapy to prevent heart attacks and osteoporosis, were found to have high risks of heart attacks, strokes, endometrial cancer, breast cancer, and rectal cancer. Nevertheless, many women still take both.[51] A whopping 23 percent of American women in their forties and fifties take antidepressants, at a higher rate than any other group by age or sex, and women are 2.5 times more likely to be taking an antidepressant than men.[52]

Common side effects of antidepressants include:

Nausea

Anxiety

Restlessness

Decreased sex drive

Dizziness

Weight gain or loss

Tremors

Sweating

Sleepiness

Fatigue

Dry mouth

Diarrhea

Constipation

Headaches

The worst side effects are increased hostility, anger, aggression, insomnia, and feelings of panic. A 2015 study reported that those taking antidepressants were "much more likely" to commit suicide.[53] As with any drug, side effects depend which one you take. Cymbalta has been linked to liver failure, Zoloft to diarrhea, Effexor to suicide, high blood pressure, and gastrointestinal bleeding.[54] Anti-depressants also seem to double the likelihood of bone fracture in menopausal women.[55]

In Italy, Effexor is commonly prescribed for hot flashes. According to Dottoressa Rossella Nappi, a gynecologist at the Centro della Menopausa all'Ospedale San Matteo di Pavia, an expert researcher into "problems women face at the end of their fertility," the practice seems to be to prescribe antidepressants not necessarily for depression, but as "off-label" drugs for women who cannot take estrogen because of prior incidences of breast tumor, endometrial cancer, melanoma, and/or thrombosis (all of the side effects brought on by hormone replacement theory and the reasons why the WHI study was abruptly stopped).[56] Dr. Nappi makes it clear, however, that antidepressants such as Effexor, or Venlafaxina, should be used only for hot flashes and night sweats, because they don't work for the "globality" of menopausal symptoms. She means they are not enough to treat "common" menopausal symptoms such as vaginal dryness and osteoporosis, to name only a few. And if you do get depressed, well, you're already covered.[57]

Another example of an off-label drug recommended by WebMD for hot flashes is Gabapentin, or Neurontin. This drug was approved to treat seizures, such as in epilepsy, but since it also seems to reduce hot flashes . . . well, why not? Again, this drug is "useful in women who can't use estrogen therapy and in those who also have migraines."

Common side effects of Gabapentin as listed by RxList:

Dizziness, drowsiness, weakness, feeling tired

Nausea, diarrhea, constipation

Blurred vision

Headache

Breast swelling

Dry mouth

Loss of balance or coordination

So while it may help your migraines, it might give you a headache. Although Gabapentin is used as a treatment for epileptic seizures, the ketogenic diet has also been proven to be an effective non-pharmaceutical treatment for epileptic seizures. The ketogenic diet is used in many hospitals and is even recognized by neurologists as the best treatment for epilepsy. Dr. Dominic D'Agostino, associate professor at the University of South Florida, is a well-known researcher into the therapeutic effects of the ketogenic diet. After reading the successful studies of the ketogenic diet for epilepsy, D'Agostino was the first to use the ketogenic diet as a way to eliminate hyperbaric oxygen toxicity, a life-threatening byproduct of breathing too much oxygen and which affects deep-water divers, such as the United States Navy Seal divers.[58]

Medications to Prevent or Treat Osteoporosis

Dr. Fuller Albright was the first to use the term "postmenopausal osteoporosis" in 1940. Albright, who had started experimenting with stilbestrol in 1938, tried to prove that estrogen stimulated osteoblasts, or bone cell growth. He came to this conclusion after his study of women who underwent oophorectomies in their twenties and early thirties showed that they often lost bone mass and developed osteoporosis before the age of forty

In his research paper, Albright and his colleagues stated, "There is considerable evidence that postmenopausal osteoporosis have a tendency to atrophy other tissues, notably the skin."[59]

However, in 1973, the FDA wrote, "There is no convincing evidence that estrogen administration reduces the loss of bone mass in aging women." It also included that, "It is possible that long-term estrogen treatment may ultimately result in decreased bone formation."[60]

In 1982, Dr. Harry Genant, a cardiologist, conducted another study, finding that women receiving a higher dose of Premarin had greater increased bone density than women on a lower dose of Premarin over a two-year span. The consensus was that Genant had confirmed Albright's hypothesis. The problem was that all of the women in his study had undergone oophorectomies, a distinction that was not included in the study. Even Genant confirmed in 2002 that he had intended his research to target women who had had their ovaries removed, not women who reached menopause naturally. "Surgical menopause brings about more abrupt and greater bone loss."[61]

Hence within two years of the FDA finally including information about the dangerous side effects of estrogen therapy this study began popping up in medical journals. Suddenly osteoporosis was understood to be a given for almost all women who would need to take preventative measures as early as their thirties, since estrogen supposedly had a protective effect. Women were duly warned of the risk of endometrial cancer, but in the 1980s, Ayerst spent most of its advertising money on images depicting women with canes or dowager's humps.

In 1984, the United States National Institute of Health convened the Consensus Development Conference on Osteoporosis. Dr. William Peck, a professor at the Washington University of Medicine in St. Louis, chaired the conference. Dr. Peck would later become a paid advisor to, among other companies, Hologic, Inc. Hologic, Inc is a developer, manufacturer, and supplier of diagnostic products, medical imaging systems, and surgical products.[62] The company's core business is diagnostics. Their website states that their products are directed at "women's health."

In 1992, WHO convened a conference in Rome with the International Osteoporosis Foundation, a nonprofit organization whose corporate advisory board consisted of thirty-one drug and medical equipment manufacturers. By the end of the conference, osteopenia was a new condition that needed treatment. It was decided that even though osteoporosis had previously been associated with the elderly, it could now endanger any woman over thirty. Osteopenia simply means bone density that is lower than normal. The problem with this is that what is normal for a fifteen-year-old will not be normal for a fifty-year-old. Doctors began telling younger and younger women that they need drugs to prevent bone deterioration. As a *New York Times* article from 2009 put it, "A diagnosis of osteopenia doesn't necessarily mean there is something wrong with you." The panel at the conference in Rome defined "normal" bone density as that of an average thirty-year-old woman.[63] Some experts argue that the formula is flawed and that it serves only to sell more drugs to treat osteoporosis.

Because there had been so much confusion since the 1992 conference, in 2009, the WHO presented an online tool called Fracture Risk Assessment Tool, or FRAX. Another article from 2009 quoted Dr. Nelson Watts, an endocrinologist and bone specialist from the University of Cincinnati, as saying, "FRAX is coming from the same people who came up with osteopenia in the first place."[64] A 2008 analysis of osteoporosis drugs in the *British Medical Journal* titled "Drugs for pre-osteoporosis: prevention or disease mongering?" concluded, "that proponents have overstated the benefits and underplayed the harms."[65]

These drugs are bisphosphonates, which were first used in the nineteenth century to soften water in irrigation systems. Bisphosphonates were studied as a treatment for osteoporosis because of their potential to reduce the loss of hydroxylapatite—the main mineral in bone and teeth formation. In the 1990s, Merck developed Alendronic acid and marketed it as Fosamax. Marketing the drug was a Merck/ Wyeth-Ayerst venture.[66] According to the *Pharma Letter,* an online publication for pharmaceutical and biotechnology news, Merck was in charge of marketing Fosamax to general practitioners and internists, while Wyeth-Ayerst was in charge of promoting the drug to gynecologists.[67] The FDA approved Fosamax to treat osteoporosis in postmenopausal women in 1995.

By 2005, bisphosphonates had become another billion-dollar business for Wyeth-Ayerst. In 2005, the *Seattle Times* published an article titled "Disease Expands Through Marriage of Marketing and Machines." "Every day in clinics and doctor's offices around the country, healthy middle-aged women slide their wrists into portable X-ray machines that calculate bone density," wrote journalist Susan Kelleher.[68] The article describes how most women walk out with a prescription for a bisphosphonate, even though doctors admit the risk of a healthy fifty-year-old getting a fracture is very low, and that millions of women in the US are wasting money and risking side effects.[69] Certainly European governments that cover these drugs are also wasting money.

In 1997, the FDA warned Merck to stop targeting all women with its Fosamax advertisements. And again in 2001, the FDA warned Merck that its Fosamax website "overstates the benefits while minimizing the risks associated with the drug."[70]

Drug companies and lobbyists created this phenomenon, again, by transforming osteoporosis into osteopenia, and by shifting the focus from treatment to prevention. It was the drug companies that created the term "osteopenia" in 1960, defined as a condition leading to osteoporosis, using measurements from bone-density machines that "the drug industry promoted, subsidized, and helped put in doctors' offices."[71] This meant companies such as Hologic, Inc.—the company that paid Dr. William Peck, chair of the NIH Consensus Development Conference on Osteoporosis in 1984—profited from not only osteoporosis, but also from osteopenia, both conditions created by a lack of nutrients.

The cost of Fosamax in 1995 ran women $600–$700 a year, for a preventative drug they were advised to take before menopause and then until they died. Ironically, studies soon showed that bisphosphonates caused osteonecrosis, which resulted in femoral breakage and caused jawbone decay. Then, in 2005, reports first surfaced that long-term Fosamax users were going to the dentist for routine dental work and ending up with broken jaws. An article in the *Journal of Endodontics* described osteonecrosis of the jaw, also known as jaw death, as a growing epidemic.[72]

By 2008, reports of unusual femoral fractures unprovoked by trauma suggested that Fosamax was actually doing more harm than good. Bisphosphonates were causing hypermineralization of bones since natural bone mineralization was inhibited. Bone tissue is made up of minerals and collagen, which together make bones tough. Osteoporosis is caused not only by a lack of minerals, but also reduced collagen. Bisphosphonates inhibit the natural turnover of mineral mass in bones, therefore reducing the bone's toughness and making it brittle. [73]

Medscape "handled" this discovery by simply suggesting that women should tell their dentists they were using Fosamax. According to an article in the *Harvard Women's Health* "News" section in 2008, Merck had promised to study its drug's effect on bone.[74] In 2006, the advice from the Merck-sponsored 2006 FLEX study, the Long-Term Extension of FIT, the Fracture Intervention Trial, seemingly in response to reports of this bisphosphonate side effect, suggested that it might be a good idea to take a break from Fosamax after five years. While I find these acronyms hilarious, I know they were specifically designed to pull the wool over the eyes of anyone bothering to read the complete study. "Flex" implies flexibility, which suggests your bones are not brittle. The problem is that many doctors find it impossible to read all these studies, and so they listen instead to the hype. By choosing cute acronyms that suggest a positive outcome for their studies, perhaps drug companies are simply trying make researchers not bother to read their studies. According to the Harvard article, bisphosphonates stay in bone tissue for years, so it is not clear if a "drug holiday" would lower the risk of osteonecrosis.[75]

Common side effects of Fosamax:

Stomach ulcer

Esophagus irritation

Nausea

Vomiting

Abdominal cramps or pain

Diarrhea

Bone pain

Fever

Chills

Muscle and joint aches

Headache

Low calcium

Digestive problems

Pain at injection site

Flu-like symptoms

Change in kidney function

Skin rash

Osteonecrosis

Medical Gaslighting

Medical gaslighting and medical gender bias influence the care women receive and how advertisers market dangerous hormone therapy to them. "Gaslighting" is a term typically used in reference to psychological abuse and is a kind of violence in which the victim is manipulated into doubting their own memory, perception, and sanity. Medical gaslighting is when a medical worker dismisses a woman's symptoms simply because she is a woman, and that her symptoms are largely caused by her emotional state; the medical worker might try to make a woman think there is nothing wrong with her. For instance, she could go to the doctor for a suspected heart attack and be sent home because she is "stressed," "menopausal," or "suffering from PMS." Of course, stress does have negative effects on a person's health, but it is not because she is a woman. If the symptoms a woman is experiencing are only associated with menopause she will be prescribed hormone therapy. Hormone therapy, whether in the form of contraception or for menopause, is dangerous. The negative side effects are the same for both. If a woman's symptoms are simply written off as caused by her reproductive organs and the reduced production of estrogen, her doctors will not look further to figure out what is causing her symptoms. Modern medicine treats symptoms with drugs and surgery, and operates as an industry. It has put menopausal women in a box that they cannot get out of to find out the real cause of why they feel bad.

In 2000, the *New England Journal of Medicine* reported that of 10,000 heart patients, (48 percent of them women) women under age fifty-five were seven times more likely to be misdiagnosed and denied care.[76] In 2016, the *Journal of the American Heart Association* reported, "Women presenting with cardiac arrest are less likely than male patients to undergo therapeutic procedures. Women are seen to be more emotional."[77]

Is this why women are twice as likely as men to be diagnosed with depression and treated with antidepressants and antipsychotics? A 2016 Danish study published in the

JAMA psychology journal in September reported that women using hormonal birth control were more likely to use antidepressants.[78] This is particularly frightening because national health services in European communities push the birth control pill on teenage girls, just as they push hormone therapy on middle-aged women, and antidepressants on women past sixty. What is even more frightening is that in1969, Harold Williams published *Pregnant or Dead* and included statistics of the spike in suicide rates in young women taking the pill. In spite of this, mechanical forms of birth control, which are equally effective and have no side effects, such as condoms and diaphragm, are never promoted.

Women were not well informed; the pharmaceutical companies made sure of that. They used the idea of liberation against women. Harold Williams, MD, blamed "the lay press, the medical press, medical organizations, drug companies, birth control enthusiasts, generally, and the Food and Drug Administration all must have a share in the blame for the delays in revealing the facts about The Pill's sorry score on safety."[79]

Barbara Seaman, whose book *The Doctor's Case Against the Pill* was a catalyst for the Nelson Pill Hearings, said, "According to the Western model, pregnancy is a disease, menopause is a disease, and even getting pregnant is a disease. Dangerous drugs and devices are given to women, but not to men—just for birth control. I've reached the conclusion that to many doctors being a woman is a disease."[80]

Gaslighting is brainwashing. How else can I explain the article written by Katie Rogers in the *New York Times* arguing for the freedom for young women to "stop their periods" with hormonal birth control?[81] The article was published in "Well," which is part of the "Health" section. The women the writer interviews all suffer from painful, or "annoying" periods. How is it that none of their gynecologists made the connection between painful menstrual symptoms and endocrine imbalance?

On the same day that this article was published, the *New York Times* printed an article about transgender men suffering from breast cancer. The doctors quoted in the article do not rule out that the hormone treatments undergone during their transition were the cause of their cancer. It does, however, state that no correlation has been found in high testosterone treatment and cancer in transgender men in Europe. Of course not. Why Europe? Because clinical trials are easier to conduct there. They are also easier to conduct in Russia.[82] Free medicine is not free. The drugs covered by national health care cost European governments a huge amount of money. In order to be able to cover the cost of medications, European governments—which are more involved in health care than the United States—must offer pharmaceutical companies preferential pricing and other subsidies for research.[83]

In 2012, an Italian newspaper bemoaned the fact that only 16 percent of Italian women chose hormonal birth control.[84] The authors stated that this was probably because women were concerned with "weight gain." The article suggests that hopefully women in Italy will get with the times and pop the pill.[85] Nowhere does it mention the numerous side effects of hormonal birth control.

Barrier Method Birth Control

Until the 1960s the diaphragm was widely used by women for birth control. Although it was promoted in the 1970s as an alternative to hormonal birth control when the women's movement raised concerns about HRT side effects, it is now seldom suggested by gynecologists, and certainly not promoted by drug companies. There is less profit in barrier birth control methods. The female condom, which was approved by the FDA in 1993, is largely ignored. Yet health organizations in developing countries promote the female condom because it gives women the right to protect themselves, not only from pregnancy, but also sexually transmitted disease.[86] The female condom still costs more than the male version (because of its lack of popularity), but the fact that it has no side effects and is more protective should make it a more publicized option for women of all ages. In 2003 Katherine O'Grady wrote that women over the age of 50 were the fastest growing group of new HIV/AIDS cases in the United States and Canada.[87] Women caring about their health, and wanting control over their bodies and their sex lives should go together.

Unfortunately, if left to the medical industry, women will have less control over their bodies. With the popularity of the pill, or shall we say, due to the marketing of the pill, the diaphragm's use plummeted. Unfortunately as of 2014 the most easily used and easily fitting diaphragm, Janssen Pharmaceuticals Inc.'s Ortho-All Flex was discontinued. Pharmaceutical companies insist that the hormonal contraception is more effective than the diaphragm. Drug companies criticize its use because it has to be inserted, and removed after eight hours. This means it has to be *properly used* to be effective. It is as effective as the male condom. Anything has to be properly used to be effective.

Women stopped using the diaphragm in the 1980s, and now young women don't even know that this type of barrier birth control exists as an option. A newer type of barrier method is available in the United States now, the FemCap, a cervical cap. There are also two other kinds of diaphragms still available in the US. Barrier methods are also a one time expense, unlike birth control pills. Women have to be fitted for them by a gynecologist, but I think the choice between that inconvenience and dangerous side effects should be an easy one.

Drugs and Their Side Effects

But medicine has known since their invention that synthetic estrogens, and too much endogenous estrogen, cause cervical cancer, breast cancer, and endometrial cancer. In fact, when scientists were developing hormone treatments—with huge financing from pharmaceutical companies—few women wanted to be a part of those studies because of the many immediate side effects of vomiting, nausea, dizziness, headaches, and stomach pain. Other side effects included bloating, mood changes, and blood clots, both for menopause and birth control trials.[88] Manufacturers and scientists chose to conduct their trials in low-income Puerto Rican birth control clinics. The doctor in charge study of the Enovid clinical trial wrote that it "gives one hundred percent protection against pregnancy [but causes] too many side reactions to be acceptable."[89] Those that could, dropped out of the studies. So the Americans then tested their pill on women in mental institutions. Schering, the German pharmaceutical giant that is now a part of Bayer, tested their hormone therapies—derived estrogen, progesterone, and testosterone—on Auschwitz prisoners. A recent modern study in 2016 did attempt a clinical hormonal birth control study on men, but it was stopped after men reported mood changing side effects.[90]

Gregory Pincus, who was part of the development team of Enovid, the first FDA-approved synthetic estrogen and progesterone birth control, had apparently tried a hormonal birth control on men, but according to Holly Grigg-Spall, in *Sweetening the Pill*, "It was rejected for men due to the number of side effects, including testicle shrinking."[91]

In her New York Times article journalist Katie Rogers argues in favor of hormonal therapy to block menstruation as a means of liberation. As does the recent advertising campaign for female hormone treatment to treat the brand new illness called "Female Sexual Dysfunction." It includes synthetic estrogen and synthetic testosterone. Women have the right to orgasm, just as they have the right to birth control, but a synthetic hormone with dangerous side effects is not the answer.

Women are led to believe they are ill, with menopause or with "Female Sexual Dysfunction," and that these drugs can fix everything. If she becomes ill from the side effects, she'll be prescribed another pharmaceutical. The idea has long been that if you fix a woman's reproductive system, you've fixed everything that is wrong with her. The discovery of hormones just made that bias easier to sell.

The fact is that medicine doesn't really listen to women's symptoms. It co-opts and humors them to get them to take a drug. According to a study called "The Girl Who Cried Pain: A Bias Against Women in the Treatment of Pain" by *Journal of Law, Medicine & Ethics*, in 2001:

"In general, women report more severe levels of pain, more frequent incidences of pain, and pain of longer duration than men, but are nonetheless treated for pain less aggressively."[92] Women's reactions were, and are, judged through a prism of hormonal change, and less importance is given to their actual symptoms.[93]

Just as high blood pressure medication works by dangerously lowering potassium levels, the medications create more side effects that will then have to be addressed by other medications. This creates a vicious circle of illness that often makes women feel as though they are in a labyrinth from which they cannot escape. We go from "Don't worry your pretty little head about it" (antidepressants), to "Cut it out" (ovaries and uterus), "Cut it off" (breasts), or "Just stop it" (synthetic or horse-derived hormones). There are other safe and efficient forms of birth control. Heavy bleeding, premenstrual pain due to endometriosis, thyroid- or blood sugar conditions, and symptoms associated with menopause can all be treated naturally. The body is so much more than its parts. Isolating a deficiency—be it hormonal or related to neurotransmitters such as serotonin—and treating the so-called deficiency with a drug does not work, and instead creates further illness.

CHAPTER FOUR

The Case for Diet

"Here I am at my advanced age, more or less walking and chewing gum at the same time. If I was a chimpanzee I would have been dead decades ago." —Kristen Hawkes [1]

Before the invention of the word "menopause," there was little confusion about about how it should be treated. The only symptom specifically associated with menopause was the cessation of bleeding. The female body was designed to do this just fine. But the longer the word has been around, the worse the symptoms get and the sooner they arrive. The stages of perimenopause and post-menopause (as if there could be a "post-menopause") have been invented to address a variety of endocrine imbalances, with the finger always pointing at a decrease in one of the three estrogen hormones, and primarily focusing on the same treatment: replacement hormones. But what if these endocrine imbalances are created by a host of other factors and are not due to the reduction of estrogen produced in the ovaries? What if the earlier onset of symptoms (perimenopause), as well as the prolongation of them (post-menopause), is really caused by something else?

"Women are the only mammalian females to live beyond their reproductive usefulness," said gynecologist Robert W. Kistner at a conference of the American College of Surgeons in 1964. "So it is by that evolutionary standard that they live too long. But since we do keep them around we should recognize that during menopause they are living in a state of hormonal imbalance, and we should treat it."[2] This was 1964, and I do not think he was kidding.

I don't think I have to explain the many levels in which Dr. Kistner was wrong. He clearly did not know much about mammals—or women. But if he was *trying* to say that the symptoms associated with menopause are caused by a hormonal imbalance . . . well, I do have to give him that one.

Of course you do want to feel healthy. Of course you want to live the longest part of your life to the fullest, but doctors, most medical researchers, and the media continue to tell you that this isn't possible without prescription drugs. Your body is a mistake. You were not supposed to live this long, and you're certainly not supposed to enjoy it. Or else, why would you be feeling this way? Something is missing, something is awry—this is the message given to women in menopause.

Something is missing, but that something is not synthetic hormones, or serotonin, or a chemical that changes how your bones regenerate. The modern woman does indeed experience menopausal symptoms. Hundreds of women called in to *The Oprah Winfrey Show* when she talked about perimenopause on April 15, 2002.[3] Women are asking their doctors for help. Doctors offer hormone therapy as a solution, but bad news about hormone therapy keeps coming. Do we still want to be at the mercy of the medical industry—just as we have been since the invention of menopause? Medicines to treat menopause are created for all women of a certain age, yet every woman is different and every body responds differently to hormonal changes. Women have different metabolisms, because of their biotype,[4] because they experience different stresses in their lives, because they have had no kids, or because they have had several. So much research has been done on how replacement estrogen would cure women of menopause, the complexity of the endocrine system has been ignored. This is surprising when you consider that back in England in 1937, Vladimir Korenchevsky and his colleagues conducted extensive research into how the adrenal hormone androstenedione affected the secretions of other glands in the endocrine system.[5]

Endocrinology is fascinating, but each new discovery led to a fixation on a single hormone, for women it was estrogen, instead of how they worked together. Each single hormone was discovered one at a time: thyroxine, one of the thyroid hormones; then insulin; then estrogen; then progesterone; and then cortisol. The entire cascade pathway of steroid hormones, which become sex hormones, and how each hormone interacts with others, creates an intricate web as delicate yet as powerful as something woven by a spider. It is called the hormone cascade because each hormone is derived from the one before it, through a complex process of synthesis, starting from cholesterol. The "hormone cascade" is the body's own system of feedback mechanisms and checks and balances. Ernest Starling understood this back in 1905, when he first coined the word "hormone." Even today, we are still a long way from isolating every hormone. While this discovery may never come to fruition, it is clear that—just as all humans need water and air—women *do* need the basic building blocks, the essentials for the creation of hormones. Of course, so do men, but that is for another book.

There are two problems facing women today: not only are more women experiencing symptoms of menopause, but for many the symptoms are also becoming more intense. At the same time, by fighting for a more balanced place in society, women are trying to regain control over the image of the menopausal woman— medicine, politics, and the arts portray them as weak, withered, and addlebrained. This dichotomy makes addressing symptoms confusing and challenging. A woman who knows that hormone replacement therapy can cause cancer, but who is beginning to experience symptoms. at the same time that her doctor starts telling her that her hormone levels are changing, is faced with a distressing set of choices. Should she take hormones to feel better, or continue to suffer? Blood tests follow. In Italy, a woman's hormone levels are tested routinely after forty-five. After forty-five, women often take it upon themselves to request testing because they feel tired, because they've put on weight, or because they've noticed changes in the texture of their skin.

In the rush to invent new medicines and surgical procedures, each somatic and psychic manifestation has been focused on locally and singularly, instead of treating the entire endocrine system. Every woman experiences menopause differently, with different symptoms, and to different degrees of intensity. This is why there are sixty-six or more symptoms of menopause. Treating healthy women with drugs that each cause their own side effects will not treat the underlying cause of the symptoms.

What is really causing the hot flashes, vaginal dryness, mood changes, sleep problems, weight gain and sagging breasts— the symptoms attributed to menopause? Yes, the production of estradiol (one of the three estrogens) is reduced, but not by much. But this is not what drives the symptoms. Menopause is an evolution designed to ensure women have a long and vibrant middle and old age. If we correct the erroneous perception that women's health issues are caused by this decline in estrogen and progesterone production, it becomes clear that the menopausal symptoms women experience are caused by something else. As we have seen, most of the body's supply of estrogen and progesterone is synthesized outside of the ovaries anyway.

Many other organs and tissues produce estradiol, including adrenal, breast, bone, vascular smooth muscle tissue, various sites in the brain, and even the skin.[6] The estrogen, or estradiol (E2), production in these sites is very high at a local level, but it needs to be synthesized. It needs to change from an androgen hormone further up the "hormone cascade," into an estrogen hormone. Ovarian estrogen is proactive, meaning it is synthesized locally by receptors at certain sites, but extragonadal estrogen is reactive, meaning it needs help from an androgen substrate (specifically C19 steroids) in order for it to be aromatized, or rendered usable for fertility.[7] The C19 steroid is a precursor to the C18 steroid, which is essentially estrogen. Excluding in the case of fertility, E2 is not necessary to bind to the many target organs and tissues where estrogen receptors are found to permit different physiological functions.

After estrogen was discovered, it was isolated and fabricated, and so it had to be put to some use. The idea of deficiency was an assumption based on a limited and prejudiced understanding of female physiology. Most medical researchers, doctors, and drug manufacturers couldn't get past the part about Darwinist procreation. Back in the 1930s, hot flashes and vaginitis were the primary symptoms associated with menopause, and this came from observational studies of women who had had hysterectomies and oophorectomies during the surgical craze of the Victorian era. As more and more receptor sites, or target organs and tissues, were discovered to which estrogens bind, a deficiency symptom for each organ and tissue was added to the list of menopausal symptoms, which grew increasingly longer. Yes, estradiol does bind to these receptors during a woman's fertile years. Yet estradiol does not begin to be produced until adolescence. After menopause, most of the estrogen essential for good health is produced in peripheral tissue, primarily the adrenal glands.

Clearly the adrenals are vital for endocrine balance. If a woman's biochemistry is functioning as it should, and estrogen (and progesterone) production is taken over by the adrenal glands and other tissues, then menopause is normally asymptomatic. Our bodies made estrogen long before the ovaries got involved (before adolescence), and we as a species have evolved to make it after menopause. The C19 steroid produced by the adrenal gland is already the component for estrogen biosynthesis in the fetus. To put it simply, if the body cannot function well without estrogen after menopause, how did it function before puberty? Are hormonal changes brought on by menopause or by cortisol and insulin levels?

Most illnesses associated with menopause—and indeed with aging—such as insulin resistance, obesity, osteoporosis, cardiovascular diseases, and reduced muscle mass, are actually caused by the reduction of steroid hormones produced in tissue other than the ovaries. They are not caused by a reduction in ovarian estradiol. After menopause, 85 percent of androstenedione—the hormone from which estrogens are synthesized—comes from the adrenal gland.[8] The body needs a lot more estrogen in order to metabolize carbohydrates. A diet high in carbohydrates and low in fat will cause insulin and cortisol levels to rise. Insulin levels rise because the pancreas will produce more insulin to lower the level of blood sugar in the blood. Insulin is a storage hormone, meaning that it makes the body hold onto fat in the fat cells. Cortisol counteracts insulin, so levels will rise in order to control insulin levels. Progesterone and estrogen counteract cortisol and insulin. Estrogen keeps insulin in check, and both progesterone and estrogen oppose the action of cortisol, and try to keep levels from going too high. This is part of the endocrine system's safety mechanism to maintain balance at any cost. High insulin and cortisol levels will create inflammation. Inflammation is the cause of all chronic disease in humans. This causes conditions as varied as diabetes, rheumatism, hypothyroidism, high blood pressure, and obesity. All of this puts the body under tremendous stress. The higher the insulin and cortisol levels, the quicker the peripheral tissues (but primarily the adrenals) will be forced to produce estrogen and progesterone in order to lower the inflammation. Then, with menopause, the production of progesterone and estrogen decrease further. This means a low-fat, high-carbohydrate diet increases menopausal symptoms.

A diet high in carbohydrates will cause a higher rate of estrogen production during a woman's fertile years. However, if a woman's adrenals are making too much estrogen in order to metabolize carbohydrates, they won't be able to keep up with demand once the ovaries reduce production. In fact, they may not be able to keep up many years before menopause. This is why many symptoms are now appearing earlier. Perimenopause is actually caused by years of a high carbohydrate diet, which forced the body to create unnatural levels of hormones. All this leads to insulin resistance, thyroid and adrenal dysfunction, and many other illnesses, such as polycystic ovary syndrome, tumors in breast, uterine, and ovarian tissue, and even cancer.

This is an imbalance that hormone therapy cannot fix. Hormone therapy is like shoving a square peg into a round hole. There is a more natural way to balance the endocrine system, even without supplements, and balancing the endocrine system is the best way to start. Much can be repaired in this way, and if some symptoms remain, the causes, can be further addressed with more specialized protocols. Achieving balance starts with the fact that the adrenals synthesize hormones from cholesterol. During menopause, your biochemistry is like a train trying to change tracks. If the other track is broken, you will experience problems; your train will be derailed. And this is exactly how menopausal symptoms can feel: going from not so bad to terrible. But menopause itself is not the underlying cause.

Let's look at the "symptoms" menopausal women are supposed to go through. We've got Suzanne Somer's seven dwarfs of menopause: Itchy, Bitchy, Sweaty, Sleepy, Bloated, Forgetful, and All-Dried-Up. It's kind of sad to see those lovable friends of fourteen-year-old Snow White renamed this way.

I say "supposed to," because, if you look at any medical website (I have researched sites in English, Italian, French, and German), you will see the same list of symptoms, perhaps with minor differences in phrasing. Depression can be lumped in with cognitive function, or it is sometimes listed separately. Here is the Mayo Clinic's list of symptoms, as of 2017:[9]

Irregular periods

Vaginal dryness

Hot flashes

Night sweats

Sleep problems

Mood changes

Weight gain and slowed metabolism

Thinning hair and dry skin

Loss of breast fullness

WebMD has a slideshow with the title, "Don't Let Menopause Ruin Your Day."[10] When I looked at WebMD three months earlier, their approach was completely different. In fact, it was scary. Either way, the end result remains the same: sending women to the doctor to get a prescription.

Their list of symptoms:

Hot flashes

Night sweats

Sleep problems

Vaginal atrophy and vaginal dryness

Low libido

Mood swings

Headaches

Thinning hair

Pimples

Brain fog

Healthline—the online subsidiary of Health on the Net foundation, and connected to the WHO—takes a different approach.[11] They list all the tissues and organs in which estrogen receptors are found, implying that only estrogen produced in the ovaries will attach to these estrogen receptors. This is misleading and insinuates that all of these places in the body will suffer from a change in estradiol, or E2, levels. But as we know, these receptors do just fine with the estrogens produced in many peripheral tissues. Healthline then lists the usual symptoms of menopause, but also throw in incontinency and frequent urination. They repeatedly use the phrase "reduced estrogen" to emphasize that because of this, misery will be your lot.

Healthline's receptor sites:

Reproductive system

Urinary tract

Heart

Blood vessels

Bones

Breasts

Skin

Hair

Mucous membranes

Pelvic muscles

Brain

What if we ignore menopause and estrogen and instead look at these symptoms one by one from a different perspective? If we examine them in this way, it becomes clear that reduced estrogen is not the cause.

Hot Flashes/Flushes/Night Sweats

This one is great for book titles. It also conveniently subverts female sexuality by turning the positive adjectival use of the word "hot," for sexy and attractive, into something negative, like sweaty and out of control. Medical websites often display stock images of women sticking theirs faces and necks directly into the airstreams of fans. They often wear orgasmic expressions. It's an odd juxtaposition: the supposedly withered woman getting turned on by the cooling air of a fan. Hot flashes are the first symptom doctors, biochemists, and pharmaceutical manufacturers attempted to address clinically with the invention of menopause. This is a vasomotor reaction, and for most women, it is first on the list when they go see the doctor. The hot flash is also a common joke. "Hot and bothered," and "hot in here," are just a couple of expressions which have been related to menopausal women. That's quite the switch from "she's hot," or "she's a hottie."

My favorite recent depiction of a hot flash in contemporary media was in Netflix's *House of Cards*. Claire Underwood, played by Robin Wright, leans into the white, cold light of the open refrigerator—a process she repeats in a few episodes, without explanation, until finally, her husband, played by Kevin Spacey, asks, "Does it hurt?" "It's not pleasant," Claire says. He asks her if there's anything that he can do and she says, "No."

All women over forty must have understood what this was referring to, but was the intelligent, gorgeous, strong, and dangerous character suffering menopausal hot flashes or was it a simply a particularly stressful time in the character's life? Was she perhaps having a vasomotor reaction to her husband's homicidal shenanigans? Incidentally, Robin Wright was forty-four when the first season of the show was released.

In her *Slate* article titled "How TV Shows Handle Menopause," June Thomas writes that they very often don't. According to Thomas, scenes like Claire Underwood's are rare. Usually, menopausal women are the butt of jokes, particularly regarding how unpleasant it would be for a man to have sex with one.[12] In the 1990s when feminist health movements were trying to get the government to provide proof about the health claims of hormone therapy, *The Cosby Show* dealt with several of the negative stereotypes surrounding menopausal women after Clair Huxtable (I have no idea why both characters share the same first name!) mentions to her children that she is entering menopause. The children joke that their mother will experience hot flashes, confusion, and crabbiness. Clair and her husband Cliff (Bill Cosby) decide to play a joke on them. Clair pretends to embody several menopausal symptoms. She snaps at her husband (mood swings), forgets her children's names (cognitive decline), weeps and then laughs maniacally (mood swings), sticks her head in the freezer and then complains that she is burning up (hot flashes). She then bursts into laughter and reveals the joke. But that was the nineties, when women were again questioning the medical interpretation of menopause.[13]

Hot flashes are a vasomotor reaction, just like blushing or breaking into a nervous sweat. Men experience them too. Remember that test you were worried about back in school? What did you feel, besides nausea and dread? Did you feel hot? Or when you ran into your first crush ? That time you got into trouble? A hot flash is a stress reaction mediated by the adrenal glands. The sympathetic nervous system is our physiological coping mechanism to stress, complicated and beautiful (as are all physiological systems in our body), and part of the fight or flight response. Many of the symptoms dumped on Ms. Menopause's front porch are adrenal reactions.

Sweating and flushing are normal adrenal reactions to stress, fear, and/or anxiety. When the sympathetic nervous system receives information from the hypothalamus as part of a fight or flight response, it will signal your blood vessels to increase blood flow to your muscle tissue so that you can run. This will also make you flush, which increases your body temperature. This, in turn, makes you sweat, which is your body attempting to control your temperature, lest you blow your top.

But why does this happen in the middle of the night, at dinner, during board meetings, or when you shake your new neighbor's hand? The body's reaction seems extreme. Where's the fire?

The problem arises because you have likely been muffling your body's natural reaction to stress for decades. For instance, your body produced excess cortisol when you stayed up all night studying for exams or those times you stayed out all night dancing. These were both stresses on your adrenal system. Working long hours, taking care of the kids on your own, even dieting to fit into that pair of jeans all wreak the same havoc and can be stressful. Maybe you ran several marathons or, like me, tirelessly studied martial arts. I remember my whole body would shake after an hour of sparring class. Of course, I knew I wasn't really in danger; there were rules in sparring, and I was never consciously afraid for my life. But what about my hypothalamus? I had to make my body think I was in danger so it would send extra blood and oxygen to my arms and legs, so that I could react quickly enough to block those punches and kicks. I hacked an adrenal reaction. When real stress situations arose with my children or my work, my sympathetic nervous system was right there. It had been trained to overreact, and quickly.

Adrenal dysfunction manifests itself in three ways, alarm, resistance, and exhaustion. Reacting at the wrong time, meaning you produce the stress hormones adrenalin and cortisol in the middle of the night (or the middle of dinner) instead of in the morning when they're supposed to gently wake you from a long, peaceful slumber. These are supposed to function as a soft pat on your shoulder to rouse you. However, when your body has produced too much cortisol over a long period of time, the gentle pat turns into nightmares, palpitations, and hot or cold sweats.

This also causes you to overreact in your daily life: for instance, you might behave as though you've just lost your job when in actuality you can't find your car keys. Conversely, you might not react at all. This is when you have exhausted your adrenals, so that they are unable to produce cortisol, and as a result, all you want to do is stay in bed.

Amazingly, you can experience all three types of reactions—to varying severity—over the course of a single day. After menopause, your adrenals take over most of your body's estrogen production, but if your adrenals are exhausted you will experience some symptoms.

Remember, this is your body's way of letting you know you need to take better care of it. Caring for your body can be annoying, but getting sick is far more frustrating. You have been reacting to low-level stress for decades, and your adrenals are tired. You were also experiencing hot flashes during your youthful fertility. All your sweat glands are activated by sympathetic fiber, the nerves that relay information back to the hypothalamus. Stressing over tests at school, promotions or difficulties at work, worrying about your kids, at any age, stresses the adrenals. Certainly that's normal, but what about the time you tried crash dieting? Did you hit the treadmill several times a week? Were you ever a vegan? It's all about the extent to which you have stressed your adrenals over the years. Here, now, in menopause, those hot flashes are your body telling you, *now*, to take care of yourself, *now*.

Doctors knew that vasomotor symptoms were an adrenal reaction back in 1924.[14] But for some reason, many doctors have forgotten this—even though hot flashes were one of the first menopausal symptoms doctors tried to treat in the 1930s. The adrenals were always involved in hot flashes. Women who had had surgical menopause had them immediately because their endocrine system was trying to catch up, to restore balance.[15] In a 2007 study, while recognizing that it is a vasomotor reaction, scientists claim, "The mechanistic role related to changes in gonadal hormones associated with VMS is not understood. Hormone therapy is the most effective treatment for VMS and other menopausal symptoms."[16]

Vaginal Dryness

For some reason, this symptom really makes me angry. Perhaps it's because this is the most feminine of menopausal symptoms. Osteoporosis can happen to men, too—but vaginal dryness? Well, that's all ours. During menopause, the vaginal tissues will supposedly atrophy so much that you will no longer be able to lubricate sufficiently for sex to be enjoyable; it will hurt both you and your partner. But the research supporting this claim was done by Dr. Robert Lewis in 1933 on young girls with gonorrhea (which attacks the mucus membranes) and on women who had had full hysterectomies.[17] Now, if you experience vaginal dryness—and experience it you will, according to the medical establishment—you can slather on a pharmaceutical lubricant which contains estrogen. Dr. John Lee even recommended natural progesterone cream for this symptom as well, since progesterone cream is transdermal and includes lubricants and skin-moisturizing agents such as shea butter and aloe vera gel. But which is the remedy, the shea butter and aloe vera gel or the progesterone?

But do women actually stop secreting vaginal mucus with menopause?

The physiology of vaginal secretion requires one essential component: stimulation. From there it gets more complex. There are actually four different kinds of vaginal lubricant, two of these are divided into subtypes. Cervical mucus glands, Bartholin's and Skene's glands, vaginal transudate, and oil and sweat glands do the secreting. These are all different kinds of vaginal lubricants. The one, and the only one that is related to fertility, is cervical mucus gland secretion. Professor Erik Odeblad, department head of medical biophysics at the University of Sweden, proved there are several types of cervical glands, or crypts, as they're also called.[18] Only one of these crypts—the S crypts—is related to the menstrual cycle, and these reduce in percentage beginning in adolescence. The mucus produced in the S crypts protect the sperm from enzymes in vaginal tissue which exist to protect the tissue from bacteria, much like intestinal tissue. The S crypt mucus safely conducts sperm through the cervix and into the uterus. As Odeblad was careful to point out, synthetic hormones, such as the pill, drastically increase the atrophy of the S crypt glands that produce mucus. Odeblad wrote that "after 3 and up to 15 months of contraceptive pill use, there is a greater loss of the S crypt cells than can be replaced."[19] His research also showed that it was the pill, the exogenous hormone, that produced this result and not a woman's natural hormone production.[20]

Essentially, there are still other glands that produce mucus and function to lubricate the vagina. Professor Odeblad spent his professional life studying the female cervix.[21] In 1962, he identified that E type (estrogen stimulated) mucus was actually made up of two types of mucin: L and S.[22] He stated that there were four types of mucin, or mucus, and that they were secreted in different areas of the cervix. The sites of secretion responded differently to hormonal stimulation. The P type of crypt increased secretion with reduced estrogen stimulation. The hormone noradrenaline, produced by the adrenals, also induces secretion from the cervical glands.

A new menopausal symptom was introduced in 2013: Genitourinary Syndrome of Menopause. In 2013, the Board of the North American Menopause Society and the International Society for the Study of Women's Sexual Health decided a term was needed for this syndrome. As a result, a terminology conference was held that same year, and they approved the new term in 2014.[23] As you will remember, this is the same North American Menopause Society founded by Dr. Wolf Utian, who received funding from Ayerst. Thus, we have a direct connection to a pharmaceutical company that stands to gain from the invention of a new syndrome.

But it is important to remember that without stimulation, there will be no secretion of any kind from any of the glands. High levels of cortisol will also prevent vaginal secretion; the adrenal glands will be busy addressing the stress caused by cortisol and will not be able to send the signals that tell the cervical glands to secrete.

As a paper on the effect of cortisol levels and genital arousal put it: "Expectations about sexual situations can reduce genital sexual arousal in men. This would be consistent with recent findings that women with high levels of anxiety showed significantly lower levels of genital arousal to an erotic film than women with moderate levels of s anxiety did. Women with high levels of chronic stress and those exposed to acute stress also show lower levels of genital arousal."[24]

Cortisol affects men too. The level of male secretion during intercourse changes with age. But late onset hypergonadism is considered very rare. As the Mayo Clinic writes in its article "Male Menopause, Myth or Reality," testosterone levels may "lower" in men, bu in women estrogen levels "plummet," and hormone therapy for men is "very controversial."[25] But men have never liked hormone therapy for themselves because of the side effects that come with it.[26]

It isn't only stress, anxiety, and nervousness that will make stimulation difficult. A high-sugar and high-carbohydrate diet will increase cortisol to the extent that it will interfere with vaginal secretion.

Sex and Libido

The beauty of menopause is that because a woman is no longer fertile, she doesn't have to worry about getting pregnant. In his book *Why Is Sex Fun?* anthropologist Jared Diamond makes the point that human bodies are designed to enjoy sex, even if not for the purposes of procreation—otherwise it wouldn't feel so good.[27] Of course, "feeling good," which involves intimacy and vaginal stimulation that produces vaginal secretion, is also related to how you feel about sex and your partner. It isn't purely mechanical. But we now know that stress will make it more difficult, mechanically, for your body to secrete vaginal fluids. When all is well, blood rushes to the male's penis and to the female's vagina when there is arousal. As explained in the last section, cortisol is very much involved in this process. With too much cortisol, your "sexual functioning," as scientific research papers put it, will be impaired. You won't be able to relax enough to have an orgasm, because orgasm requires the involvement of the central nervous system to feel the sensual experience. Too little cortisol and you won't be able to stay awake. Sexual response measures are actually the same for men and women. Not only is performance (erection in men, swelling and lubrication of the vaginal tissue in women) reduced when there are high or low cortisol levels, but so is the ability to react or respond to stimuli. Women who had a high-functioning sexual response (meaning they achieved orgasm) had lower cortisol levels during sex, whereas women who were sexually abused in the past experienced an increase in cortisol during sex and a lower sexual response.[28] Since, according to a research paper from 2011, only 8 percent of all women have vaginal orgasms (without clitoral stimulation), it seems that tactile stimulation of the clitoris will increase the response of the female central nervous system. However, this sort of stimulation won't work if your sympathetic nervous system is busy worrying about danger. And if your cortisol level is high, your sympathetic nervous system will automatically assume you're in danger; remember, the purpose of cortisol is to help you escape.

Cognitive Changes

When medical writers describe cognitive changes that may occur during menopause, they are referring to problems with mood and memory. In 1996, Kuiper, et al., discovered the estrogen receptor beta (ER-β) in the prostate and ovarian tissue of rats.[29] Shortly thereafter, researchers discovered tissue distribution of estrogen beta receptors in neuron clusters throughout the brains of mice, meaning that estrogen was needed to bind to these receptors for optimal brain function. Before long, it was discovered that the brain synthesizes its own quantity of estradiol, also the C19 aromatase enzyme, but that a reduced quantity of estradiol (E2) was associated with diseases such as Alzheimer's and Parkinson's. Furthermore the number of estrogen receptor alpha receptors were seen to decline, not only in the female uterus but also in the hypothalamus.[30]

Clearly this must present a problem for women, meaning here was yet another deficiency to be addressed. Not only would women feel less womanly—because estrogen is what causes the development of breasts and curves during puberty—but even their brains would be affected. That dizzy dame, who gets confused and drops things? Well, that's because of her menstrual cycle! Low estrogen is associated with "brain fog" during a woman's cycle.

WebMD posts: "Some experts believe that some women are more vulnerable to the menstrual cycle's normal changes in estrogen. They suggest it's the roller coaster of hormones during the reproductive years that create mood disturbances,"[31] and that estrogen has an effect on the parts of the brain that "control emotion.[32] It does state that none of this has been proven. However, the article mentions that postpartum depression is associated with a drop in estrogen levels and that some studies show perimenopausal depression can be alleviated by taking transdermal estrogen. Yet the same research has also shown that estrogen therapy does not help treat depression in postmenopausal women.

At the first Women's Brain Health Academic Symposium in Toronto, Gillian Einstein, professor of psychology and public health at the University of Toronto, discussed how stress affects women and their cognition. "Humans are in a world," she explains, "they're living in stressful circumstances and different gendered environments. These environments affect human biology."[33]

"I want women to be circumspect about the effect of their hormones on their mood and cognition," said Einstein. "It may or may not be PMS that makes you grumpy. It's possible that your husband really did do something crappy, and you have a reasonable response to it."[34] Yet so far, the majority of women's health research has focused on reproductive health, rather than on such systems as the nervous, musculoskeletal, cardiovascular, and immune systems and the ways in which they might be influenced by hormones like estrogen. In truth, different forms of estrogen act on different parts of the body. The estradiol that is supposedly missing due to menopause is synthesized in the brain. One form, 17beta-estradiol, is made in the ovaries and has reproductive functions. The other, 17alpha-estradiol, is made in the brain.[35]

Brain Fog

So why is Brain Fog now accepted as a symptom of menopause? How is this different from the brain fog that is an accepted symptom of PMS, when women are at their peak of fertility? Doctors also lump Alzheimer's and depression into the list of possible menopausal symptoms and often recommend medication. We go from dizzy in fertility to confused in menopause. In 2012, the University of Rochester Medical Center published an article titled "'Brain Fog' of Menopause Confirmed." The article mentions a study with the University of Chicago that analyzed the brain function of seventy-five women in their forties and fifties and came to the conclusion that menopausal brain fog was real. The lead researcher, Miriam Weber, a neuropsychologist at the University of Rochester Medical Center, is even quoted as saying, "If a woman approaching menopause feels she is having memory problems, no one should brush it off or attribute it to a jam-packed schedule."[36] Why not brush it off as a jam-packed schedule and due to stress?

Brain fog—that head in the clouds feeling, that "I went into a room and forgot what I came in here for" feeling—is also a symptom of hypothyroidism, adrenal fatigue, and diabetes. This is why balancing the entire endocrine system is so important, rather than focusing exclusively on estrogen.

Of course, this news was picked up and published in the Daily Mail UK, and the Huffington Post. WebMD published the study in 2016 with the headline: "More Evidence Menopause 'Brain Fog' Is Real."[37]

The University of Rochester study found memory skills tend to drop as estrogen levels dip at ages forty-five to fifty-five. Julie Dumas, an associate professor of psychiatry at the University of Vermont, was interviewed for the article, and possibly in an attempt to console women of the age in question, said, "There really is something going on in the brain. You're not crazy."[38]

Lower estradiol levels "seemed key" to changes in brain activity. But Dumas also said hormone replacement therapy was not the answer. "There's no good evidence that it benefits the brain," she said.[39] "No one is prescribing estrogen for women's brains," Dumas said in a *U.S. News & World Report* follow-up article, investigating the issues with the research.[39]

Dr. JoAnn Pinkerton, executive director of the North American Menopause Society, said, "In the absence of more definitive findings, hormone therapy cannot be recommended at any age to prevent or treat a decline in cognitive function, or dementia."[40]

For the University of Rochester study, seventy-five women were tested for their ability to learn and retain new information, to mentally manipulate new information, and to sustain their attention over time. They were also asked about some of the other "seven dwarfs of menopause": depression, anxiety, hot flashes, and problems sleeping. Women who complained of depression and hot flashes were also more likely to have memory problems. The study did not connect memory problems to estrogen levels. Lower hormone levels did not mean more memory problems. So then why was the study even published as relating to menopause? Perhaps because it was first published in the *Journal of the North American Menopause Society*, the organization of Dr. Wulf Utian. Pfizer, which inherited Wyeth-Ayerst's line of products, and which makes billions of dollars in revenue from hormone replacement therapy, teamed up with the University of Rochester to develop new drugs to treat menopausal. In 2004, the University of Rochester signed a license agreement with Pfizer. In this way the drug giant could use the University of Rochester patent developed by the neurology department for a non-hormonal drug Pfizer had in development to combat hot flashes.[41] At the same time, *Business Wire* reported that "Millions of women have stopped taking hormone replacement as a result" of the WHI study linking hormone replacement therapy to cardiovascular disease and breast cancer.[42] In 2002, before safety questions dampened sales, sales of hormone replacement drugs topped $3 billion, and the hormone replacement drug Premarin (made by Pfizer) was the third-highest selling drug in the US.[43]

An article on the site BrainHQ called "The Brain on Menopause" asks: "Do you feel like you've been forgetting more often or having trouble concentrating? A lot of women notice cognitive changes during menopause that leave them feeling "fuzzy," a little (or a lot) less sharp than they used to be. For many women, these are troubling changes. They wonder—and worry about—where it will end?"[44] This is followed by the statement: "It's not entirely clear why these symptoms arise during menopause."[45] All of the research articles, websites, and newspapers conclude on a similar note, telling readers that scientists cannot prove their theories because the brain (and estrogen activity) is complicated. The University of Rochester study measured estradiol levels and follicle-stimulating hormone. They found no connection between their levels and memory problems, but they attempt to make a connection between decreased ovarian estradiol levels and brain fog. The website BrainHQ—which states that it is in partnership with clinicians, researchers, and universities—offers brain exercises, but explains that "part of the logic behind hormone replacement therapy was that it might help prevent such cognitive changes." It concludes the article by saying diet and exercise are also important.[46]

Sleep Problems

Insomnia is considered a major symptom of menopause. Sleep problems and mood swings are lumped together with cognition, but the brain isn't the only thing that affects sleep. Many women have a hard time getting to sleep when they are premenstrual, and some more recent research papers grant that insomnia will affect memory and mood.[47] Unable to sleep? You'd better watch out for Somer's seven dwarfs, as you're likely to become bitchy, weepy, sleepy, and forgetful. Endocrine balance has a crucial role in how well we sleep, how easily we fall asleep and stay asleep, and whether or not we wake up feeling refreshed. This is the physiological purpose of sleep: it gives us a chance to rest, to restore, and to regenerate.

Having trouble falling asleep and having trouble staying asleep affect more women than men. Sleep problems can increase with age, but is that because of the decrease in the body's estrogen? As we know, estradiol production starts to decline in the fetus, so that isn't the answer. The rate of insomnia is increasing. Scientists have done huge amounts of research. People go to sleep clinics to learn why they are having trouble sleeping and what they can do to fix it. Studies show that insomnia affects poor people more than rich people. It is a major symptom of post-traumatic stress disorder. Doctors agree that stress triggers insomnia, and one study concluded that there "seems to be an association between depression, anxiety, and insomnia."[48] Insomnia is on the rise in the United States, and in Italy, the insomnia rate has doubled in the last five years.[49] The architecture of sleep is a complex construction of hormones and neurotransmitters. Since different elements make for good sleep hygiene, we cannot blame reduced estrogen levels. Sleep disorders would seem to be caused by a cortisol imbalance.

Circadian rhythms influence sleep-wake cycles, hormone release, body temperature, and other important bodily functions. Normal sleep involves different cycles: one light, another deeper slow-wave sleep, and the deeper REM sleep, then finally deeper stage of sleep is marked by another transition between light sleep and even deeper sleep. The light sleep cycle moves from wakefulness to sleep, taking about 10 minutes. The next stage lasts about 20 minutes, and it is during this stage that body temperature decreases and the heart rate slows down. It can take 30 minutes before REM sleep is reached. Here, the brain starts to dream. Eye movements are rapid and the brain is active. REM is also called "paradoxical sleep," because even though the brain is active, the muscles are in a state of almost complete paralysis. This is one of the reasons why REM sleep is restorative. The brain shrinks during REM sleep, allowing for cerebrospinal fluid to flush out toxins.[50] The hormone melatonin maintains the circadian rhythm, which can be disturbed by cortisol spikes due to stress or high insulin levels.

Although insomnia is considered a menopausal symptom, much of the research into insomnia is done on age-related insomnia. "With aging, the production of melatonin declines and is shifted to later hours while the production of cortisol increases and its peak occurs earlier in the night."[51] Researchers found that cortisol was to blame for disturbing the sleep of the insomnia sufferers they studied, and one paper stated, "The clinical benefit from a decrease in cortisol during the early part of the night may lie beyond the improvement of sleep into a better control of blood pressure, metabolism, and mood."[52]

A 2013 study in *Sleep Medicine Reviews* describes the function of the cortisol awakening response (CAR), which rises rapidly after waking, following the circadian rhythm. After waking, cortisol levels increase by as much as 75 percent, peaking approximately thirty minutes after a person wakes up. The authors conclude that the function of the CAR may be related to arousal, energy boost, and/or anticipation, and suggest that an imbalance in the cortisol awakening response could cause daytime dysfunction and cause insomnia.[53] Balancing your cortisol level and paying attention to how your adrenals respond to stress will benefit the quality of your sleep.

Mood Swings

Ups and downs, highs and lows, joy is fleeting, despair eternal. Maybe you think of yourself as an emotional or unstable person; maybe you've always felt this way or maybe this is a new feeling. Drug companies rely on women feeling unstable or experiencing mood swings. The reason we feel this way is because, in order to keep the endocrine system stable, women require a certain amount of fat in our diet, and fat has been maligned for over six decades. Women have been consuming less and less fat, or even none at all.

The neurotransmitters serotonin, dopamine, and norepinephrine are essential for a balanced endocrine system. Hormone imbalances affect your brain chemistry, as well as the chemistry of your second brain, the gut. Take sugar, for example. Sugar stimulates the same neurotransmitters as cocaine and heroin. Sugar increases cortisol levels, which causes you to feel nervous, and once those sugar levels crash, you feel depressed. By removing sugar and carbohydrates from your diet, you can fix this rollercoaster ride.

But cholesterol levels also play a role in the depression women experience. A Swedish study in 1998 found that middle-aged women with low cholesterol were more likely to suffer from depression.[54] Fat makes neurotransmitters stick to receptor sites, and it works to deliver those neurotransmitters to specific protein receptors. Low-fat diets will inhibit the release of mood neurotransmitters, such as dopamine and serotonin.[55] You need fat to be happy and tranquil, and low-fat diets cause depression in women.[56]

Weight Gain and Slowed Metabolism

In a 2012 study in the journal *Climacteric*, researchers came to the conclusion that although "weight gain per se is attributed to the menopause transition, the change in hormonal milieu at menopause is associated with an increase of total body and an increase in abdominal fat."[57] The study concludes that "there is strong evidence that estrogen and estrogen-progestin therapy may partly prevent this menopause-related change in body composition."[58] The same sentence also states that insulin sensitivity was improved by estrogen therapy. If there is too much insulin weight will be gained because insulin tells the body to hold onto fat, or energy, in the form of fat molecules in cells. The best way to improve insulin sensitivity is by reducing stress and by reducing carbohydrates in the diet, since high insulin and cortisol levels are what create insulin resistance in the first place. Increased weight gain would seem to be attributed to other factors, and not the decreased level of ovarian estradiol production. Taking a synthetic hormone to prevent weight gain doesn't make sense if insulin sensitivity is the issue.

Researchers have tried very hard to prove that reduced estrogen levels produce negative effects. After the writers of a 2010 paper in *Journal of Steroid Biochemistry and Molecular Biology* state that high insulin levels have been associated with obesity and inflammation since 1953, they go on to postulate that "manipulation of gonadal steroid levels can influence leptin and insulin sensitivities and body fat distribution."[59] There is an easier way. Balancing the endocrine will improve insulin sensitivity. Why not just improve insulin sensitivity with diet? Wouldn't that be a better treatment, as there are no side effects?

A research paper in *Diabetes* makes it clear that estrogen will increase weight gain in menopausal women, because of estrogen's effect on fatty acid storage and oxidation,[60] yet researchers writing in a different issue of *Climacteric* insist that, "here is strong evidence that estrogen therapy may partly prevent this menopause-related change in body composition and the associated metabolic sequelae. However, further studies are required to identify the women most likely to gain metabolic benefit from menopausal hormone therapy in order to develop evidence-based clinical recommendations."[61]

The researchers are clearly trying very hard to make weight gain a menopausal symptom, and after all their research, they come to the conclusion that "the effect of low estrogen on increased obesity has been linked to estrogen receptor alpha," the estrogen receptor found in the brain.[62]

Or is it the effect of high cortisol. Elissa S. Epel, lead investigator who conducted a study at Yale's psychology department, said, "Greater exposure to life stress or psychological vulnerability to stress may explain their enhanced cortisol reactivity. In turn, their cortisol exposure may have led them to accumulate greater abdominal fat."[63]

Historically, heavier women were associated with menopausal symptoms. The Byzantine emperor Justinian I's personal doctor wrote that menopause begins early in some women, especially those who are "very fat." In twelfth century Salerno, a female physician wrote the *Book on the Conditions of Women*, one of three texts that make up the *Trotula*. When describing menstruation in it Trota writes that "a purgation of this sort usually befalls women about the 13th or 14th year or a little later according to whether heat or cold abounds in them more." Menstruation, she wrote, "lasts up to about the 50th year if she is lean; sometimes up to the 60th or 65th year if she is moist; in the moderately fat up to about the 45th." Historically obesity—today seen as a symptom of metabolic disorder, associated with diabetes and endocrine imbalance—caused early menopause, not the other way around.

Loss of Breast Fullness (also known as saggy breast syndrome)

Breasts develop in adolescence so that we may nurse our young. "Perky" breasts are associated with ovarian estrogen levels. According to Google's Ngram Viewer, the phrase "perky breasts" has been in use since 1950, but soared in the year 2000. In a *Cosmopolitan* advice column from 2014, a reader asks "How Important Are Perky Boobs?" Admirably, the advisor, Ms. Hill, responds, "You get two breasts. And it's useless to worry about what might turn on a guy a bit more or less, because the only way to change that is plastic surgery, which generally fucking sucks, aesthetically and medically. So let me quote the children's book *Pinkalicious*: 'You get what you get and you don't get upset.' You get *your* breasts, not anybody else's. That's it. No returns."[64]

Unfortunately, a year later, Cosmopolitan published an article titled "5 Ways to Make Your Chest Look Perkier."[65]

In 2011, the *Guardian* ran an article about Britain's soaring rates of breast reconstruction, quoting a British plastic surgeon. He said there was too much emphasis on the health risks of breast implants, and, "It's always slightly unreasonable for a man to lecture a woman about the benefits of being feminine, but if you have no breasts or completely empty breasts I'm told you don't feel feminine, there can be self confidence issues. There's a perception that women having breast implants are all bobble-headed bimbos looking for enormous pneumatic breasts, but this is not the case. They are ordinary women."[66]

Cancer as a side effect is the growing concern about breast implants and surgery to render breasts more "perky." Who told this surgeon that women don't feel feminine with "completely empty" breasts? And what does "completely empty" even mean? Empty of what? What happened to saggy?

The plastic surgeon tells the journalist that it isn't throngs of "young women seeking to emulate glamour models"[67] requesting his expertise, but postmenopausal women in their fifties and sixties. So we learn that it's due to menopausal women with empty breasts that breast reconstruction rates are soaring. They don't have to spell it out, but it is seems clear that the plastic surgeon is associating "empty breasts" with estrogen deficiency. Clearly hormone therapy does not work for this menopausal symptom if surgery is required.

But it just isn't true. Menopause does not cause breasts to sag. You hit forty-five and your breasts don't just deflate. But then again, women are *also* taught that breastfeeding will cause their breasts to sag. I'm reminded of the 1990 movie *Revenge,* starring Kevin Costner, Anthony Quinn, and Madeleine Stowe. Anthony Quinn won't let his wife (played by Madeleine Stowe) get pregnant, because he thinks it will spoil her looks. Damned if you do, damned if you don't.

In the 1970s Nestlé was criticized for marketing its baby formula to mothers in developing countries. Because of the marketing, many African women did not breast feed their babies. One of the results was that poor women diluted the breast milk to save money, and many malnourished infants died.[68] I won't go checking into Nestlé milk formula donations to plastic surgery research journals (not yet anyway).

What is it that causes a loss in breast "fullness" or "density," as researchers like to call it? It isn't estrogen. Research from 2016 demonstrated that adolescent girls with diets high in saturated fat had a higher breast density ratio than adolescent girls who consumed less saturated fat and more mono- and polyunsaturated fat (vegetable oil).[69] Every single cell membrane should be made up of at least 50 percent saturated fat. Saturated fat is what makes skin cells elastic, resistant, and strong. If the cells are denied healthy fat, or stuffed with mono- or polyunsaturated trans fat, skin cells will become more easily damaged. On a high-fat diet, breasts become fuller.

Another recent study found that dietary fat reduced skin aging in Japanese women. Facial wrinkles, such as crow's feet, were measured with the Daniell scale. The researchers came to the conclusion that higher dietary fat was associated with increased skin elasticity.[70]

So what happens during the surgery to restore fullness to one's breasts? The plastic surgeon cuts around the nipple and makes an anchor shape down the front (a proportionally larger or smaller anchor depending on breast size), inserts the implants, then removes the anchor triangle, closes the flaps, repositions the nipple, and sews it all back up. Apart from being invasive and leaving some scars, this somewhat barbaric solution will not last; the implants may have to be replaced after a number of years. More importantly, reduced breast fullness was actually caused by lack of elasticity. But as Dr. Eisenberg helpfully explains in an article entitled Do Breast Implants Need to Be Replaced Every 10 Years from 2015 in the press release distribution service *Marketwired*, "Like breast implants, your refrigerator comes with a warranty, but you don't automatically replace it when that warranty expires. You'll probably keep it until it breaks down, unless you are redoing your kitchen and want a bigger or smaller model."[71]

Besides possible cancer due to a reaction to the material used in breast implants, there is the risk of another side effect due to this breast surgery, for enhancement or for reconstruction. Increasing numbers of women are choosing to undergo breast reconstruction surgery after preventative mastectomies. These women are finding that breast reconstruction leaves them with numb breasts. A *New York Times* article described that the up-to-date medical technology "using a woman's belly fat to create the new breast, sparing the nipple, minimizing scarring with creative incisions and offering enhancements like larger, firmer lifted breasts" falls short of what these women were led to believe. The article says that the new "nipple-sparing surgery has yet to fulfill its promise, and in most cases, sensation is not restored."[72] The point I am making is that menopausal women are made to feel they should have breast surgery in order to enjoy "enhancements like larger, firmer lifted breasts" because their ovaries are producing a reduced amount of estrogen.

Osteoporosis

Osteoporosis as a menopausal symptom is one of the most lucrative developments in the modern medical "treatment" of menopause. Women in the United States and Europe are instructed to get bone density tests once they are menopausal. In Italy, hundreds of thousands of women over fifty-two receive letters in the mail, courtesy of ASL (the Italian national health service), instructing them to get a Mineralometria Ossea Computerizzata (MOC), or densitometry exam, every year. More than this, many women's health websites advise starting much earlier due to the risks associated with the recently invented peri-menopause. In Italy, however, this test is not covered before fifty-two years of age. [73]

WebMD says, "There is a direct relationship between the lack of estrogen during perimenopause and menopause and the development of osteoporosis." According to the medical establishment, 50 percent of women over fifty suffer from osteoporosis. They further claim that more than 75 percent remain undiagnosed. Osteoporosis brings with it fragile bones and the risk of spontaneous fractures—hence the necessity for "menopausal women to get bone mineral density testing, also known as bone densitometry. Bone mineral density testing is the gold standard for diagnosing osteoporosis in certain bones."[74]

Humanitas Salute—the Italian version of the Mayo Clinic website—describes the gold standard bone densitometry test as a noninvasive screening done by X-ray. It tests the mineral density of the lumbar spine, the vertebra, and the femora, and each exam costs forty-eight euro.[75]

Despite the insistence that women over thirty-five are at risk of osteoporosis, many research papers demonstrate that osteoporosis is a multi-factorial condition that is more related to dietary deficiency and hormonal imbalance.[76] A paper from February 2017 investigated the association between the peripheral skeleton-predicted failure load (how much weight a bone can stand without breaking) and stiffness, bone microstructure, and dietary protein intakes from various origins (animal—divided into dairy and nondairy—and vegetable origins) in healthy postmenopausal women. The researchers concluded that the results "indicate that there is a beneficial effect of animal and dairy protein intakes on bone strength and microstructure, that bone mineral density was higher in the peripheral bone structure of women who ate animal protein."[77] Furthermore, younger women are suffering from vitamin D deficiency—not because of lack of sunlight, but because of low-fat diets.

So what leaches the minerals from bones? Nutritional deficiency is a major factor. Having many children, for one—and therefore experiencing prolonged lactation—uses lots of nutritional energy. The density of the lumbar spine and the femoral neck was significantly reduced in women who had multiple children. Researchers also concluded that "Multiparity and prolonged lactation have negative impact on BMD especially within a socioeconomic group whose nutritional intake is borderline."[78]

Inflammation and increased cortisol levels also play a large role. "Findings of the present study implicate a role for cytokine pattern-mediated inflammation in patients with osteoporosis is another contributing factor in developing osteoporosis."[79]

While cortisol levels are typically increased by stress, Dr. Yudkin, British physician and author of *Pure, White, and Deadly*, found that eating too much sugar also increased cortisol levels.[80] Bones are made up of 65 percent mineralized collagen, which gives bones their solid infrastructure, and of 35 percent collagen tissue which is shaped like a crisscrossed protein similar to a beehive.[81] Vitamin D is essential for collagen production. A high-carbohydrate diet leaches the minerals necessary for collagen and bone formation, and a low-fat diet inhibits Vitamin D3 synthesis—

also imperative for bone density.81 A dietary approach to improving bone density would seem to be a sounder method for reducing the risks of osteoporosis.

Women—and their doctors—are led to believe that the research linking osteoporosis to menopause is sound. Yet a Canadian study from 2016 analyzed all of the papers on osteoporosis from 2009 to 2012 and found that most involved researchers who had ties to companies with pharmaceutical companies.82

Cortisol and Stress

William Buchan was a seventeenth-century British scholar and mathematician, who in 1769, published his book *Domestic Medicine; or, the Family Physician*. In it Buchan distinguished menopause from amenorrhea, and argued that menopause preserved the health of older women. He also emphasized healthy living for all women, suggesting that poor diet and a lack of exercise and fresh air could cause digestive and nervous issues. He advised against using drugs to bring on menstruation. "I think the administration of medicine always doubtful, and often dangerous, and would much rather teach men how to avoid the necessity of using them, than how they should be used."83

Cortisol has a profound effect on our entire biology. It affects our endocrine system, which, as we know, produces all our hormones: including the thyroid hormone (which regulates metabolism); insulin (which regulates blood sugars and stores fat); and our sex hormones (estrogen, progesterone, and testosterone, which regulate sexual function, menstrual cycles, and menopause). Cortisol affects our digestion and our immune system, and it suppresses neurotransmitters—the brain chemicals that determine energy, mood, mental clarity, focus, and sleep. Cortisol cues our body to hold onto body fat, so this means it plays a huge role in weight gain. It is also a major contributor to anxiety and depression. When our cortisol levels are optimal, we feel mentally sharp, clear, and motivated. When our cortisol levels are off, we tend to feel foggy, listless, and fatigued. The vasoconstriction due to high cortisol levels reduces blood circulation to the lungs, muscles, bones, and even skin and hair. High or low cortisol is associated with all of the symptoms we have discussed, from vaginal dryness to osteoporosis. The symptoms associated with adrenal dysfunction, particularly in Cushing's syndrome, which is caused by clinically high levels of cortisol in the body, are the symptoms nearly identical to those associated with menopause.[84]

Common symptoms for Cushing's syndrome:

Thin skin, tissue atrophy

Facial hair in women

Osteoporosis

Excess sweating

Mood swings—such as being more irritable, depressed, or anxious than usual

Lowered libido

Obesity

High blood pressure

Frequent urination

Cushing's syndrome is caused by the adrenal glands over producing cortisol. It has historically been associated with congenital deformation of the adrenals or with adrenal tumors that cause hypercorticism, when the adrenal cortex secretes an excess of cortisol. Pituitary Cushing's occurs when a benign tumor in the pituitary gland causes an excess of ACTH, the hormone that stimulates the adrenal cortex to produce cortisol. This excess can also be medically induced by lengthy treatment for asthma, rheumatism, and immunosuppression. Cortisone was the wonder drug that came after estrogen. But by the 1960s, the toxic side effects stemming from overuse were well documented. Warnings were issued, but cortisone still remains the standard treatment for asthma, and for joint, muscle, and skin inflammation.

The unnatural amount of estrogen in contraceptives and hormone therapy can cause pseudo-Cushing's syndrome, which is a name given to different states which have the same clinical features as Cushing's syndrome, basically anything that puts the body's biochemistry under so much stress that excess cortisol is produced. Estrogen excess from hormone therapy or from excess carbohydrates is the reason Cushing's syndrome occurs more prevalently in middle-aged women. Women are three times more likely to develop a cortisol-secreting adrenal tumor. The symptoms listed for menopause and Cushing's syndrome are so similar that Medscape emphasizes the importance of a differential diagnosis between menopause and pheochromocytoma.[85] Because it tries to control excess cortisol, estrogen are two of the delicate strands of the endocrine web that balance with cortisol and insulin in the negative feedback loop. Lowering insulin and cortisol levels will restore the balance.

The blame has been laid on estrogen. Too much gives you PMS, too little gives you menopause. But it is really the other hormone—cortisol—which is causing menopausal symptoms. Cortisol serves an important function. You can't live without it, but too much puts your body in a state of alarm, an incessant catabolic state, much like being on fire. Changing how you eat puts the fire out. Can it really be that simple? Yes. It may take some time and some coaxing, but by balancing your blood sugar and lowering your cortisol levels, you will begin feeling the benefits in just a few days.

CHAPTER FIVE

Fat For Balance

"You'll calm down when you get to be about fifty," said the female psychotherapist to the young woman suffering from mood swings, depression, bulimia, and alcohol and drug cravings.

Doctor . . .

Menopause makes us live longer. With a balanced endocrine system, it slows all physiological aging.[1] We have evolved to transition elegantly from fertility to infertility, without all the storms that come in the form of symptoms.

If menopause is a good thing, too much estrogen is a bad thing. It not only causes high cortisol, but a host of other maladies—the worst of which is cancer. The endocrine system requires constant balance to function, with constant communication and feedback between the autonomous nervous system, different hormone-secreting glands, and the receptors that bind to the hormones. The sympathetic nervous system is your fight or flight mode; it's what turns up the cortisol, sends blood and oxygen to the muscles, raises your blood pressure, cools you down with sweat, makes your heart beat faster, signals the liver to make glucose so you can react faster and run. The parasympathetic nervous system relaxes you. This is when our heart rate returns to rest: we can digest; we can make love. Our bodies know that life is like walking a tightrope, and we walk it every day, suspended over the unknown, in perfect balance between the sympathetic and parasympathetic nervous systems. Synthetic hormones and a high-carbohydrate diet, however, raise estrogen levels and confuse, block, and damage that balance. So if feel you have menopausal symptoms your endocrine system is probably wobbling, trying to right itself.

Do you remember Weebles, the self-righting toys that came out in 1971? At nine, I was perhaps too old for them, but I remember the catchphrase: "Weebles wobble, but they don't fall down." Think of your endocrine system like a Weeble, working hard to keep you standing upright, despite the onslaught of stress that feels like it is trying to push you down. Our "wobbling" is caused by the stress reaction produced by the adrenals. High cortisol and high blood sugar are normal reactions to stress; problems arise when these levels are consistently high. Mess too much with the endocrine system and you might fall down. Falling down is getting very sick.

Fat is what keeps you up; the fat you eat keeps your body stable. It turns off the cortisol reaction and bridges the gap between the sympathetic and parasympathetic nervous systems. Just look at what fat does for the body: it makes cells grow and creates new ones; it organizes them into tissues and organs; it activates adrenalin; turns on the immune system and turns off autoimmune reactions; it synthesizes serotonin; eliminates toxins; and it makes adrenal cortex hormones, thyroid hormones, testosterone, estrogen, and vitamin D.

Eating good fat is a simple way to reset the whole system of communication between the hypothalamus, the pituitary, the thyroid, the adrenals, the pancreas, the ovaries, and the uterus. It allows you to get back to all the benefits of menopause and causes no side effects. This means burning it, metabolizing it, and allowing the body to use it the way we evolved to. In other words, we must consume the very thing we've been told to avoid like the plague for the last sixty years. Are we any healthier for refusing to eat fat? No. Not only has chronic illness of all kinds skyrocketed, but "menopause" has worsened. Women today are sicker, even though they dutifully follow orders to exercise, avoid saturated fat, eat their fruits and vegetables, and undergo all the various tests to alert them if none of that is working. Mammograms? Breast cancer is rising. In the United States, healthy women are having mastectomies because their mothers had breast tumors. Colonoscopies? In the US, colon cancer is the second leading cause of death among women, with 70 percent of these women over the age of fifty. Heart disease? In the US, heart disease claims one in four women. In Italy, around one thousand cases of cancer are discovered every day. Avoiding fat is not working.

We have to go back—back to before estrogen was ever discovered. Back before surgeons routinely cut out women's uteri and ovaries, past the nineteenth-century English doctors who realized that those women who worked long hours in dark places and gave birth to many children were getting cancer at higher rates than women living in the country. We have to go back to before humans picked up the hoe and the sickle. Before the female endocrine cycle— that complex web of fat-soluble hormones—was altered.

Agriculture provides a great deal of carbohydrates. Before this, women consumed carbohydrates only in the form of wild greens, some fibrous tubers, and the occasional handful of berries. Female hunter-gatherers breastfed longer, and because breastfeeding suppressed ovulation, they had children about four years apart, which allowed for more time between pregnancies. But with the introduction of carbohydrates as a dietary staple, estrogen levels rose, which meant that women in agricultural societies began having more children.[2] Children were given carbohydrate-heavy food in the form of mashed grain. This in turn brought on menstruation at a younger age, and so women began having children at a younger age.

As food changed, so too did the female body. With the diet now higher in carbohydrates, bones moved and tilted. The pelvic cavity narrowed,[3] the female body shrunk,[4] the hips changed shape,[5] and the fetus grew heavier and fatter.[6] All of this made delivery more painful and far more dangerous. Archeologists have found few skeletons of newborn babies among the human remains of early hunter-gatherer groups,[7] but with the advent of agriculture, more infants died. Anthropological studies show that when humans introduced sugary carbohydrates into their diet, their health suffered. Ancient Egyptians, for instance, had rotten teeth and osteoporosis. Native American tribes in the American Southwest, who ate more corn and agave, had rotten teeth and osteoporosis.[8]

Today we associate food that is sweet with gratification. All our lives, we've been rewarded and consoled with sugary and carbohydrate-laden foods; this means that when times are tough, or after a stressful day, these are the foods we've been programmed to turn to. But this has not always been the case. In hunter-gatherer societies, fat was the most valued part of the animal. Labor in hunter-gatherer societies was less divided. Women hunted and men gathered. Aboriginal Chipewyan women from Canada in charge of rabbits snaring, paused their work to cook a rabbit for a meal.[9] Studies of Paleolithic skeletons in South Africa showed that women and men had similar collagen and bone composition.[10] Women were healthier in the Paleolithic era. Signs of anemia, dental caries, and osteoporosis start to show up in women in the Neolithic era, in agricultural societies. Labor became more divided with the advent of agriculture.

In "The Space Crone," Ursula K. Le Guin said that women have to give birth to themselves during menopause.[11] She has a point. In the womb, we enjoy a rich brew of fatty acids essential to our development, and breast milk continues to provide this fatty liquid until we are weaned. Babies who are breastfeeding are in ketosis, the metabolic state in which the body burns fat instead of glucose for energy. We need to take care of ourselves the way we evolved to, and by consuming fat—not transfats—we not only give birth to ourselves, but also restore ourselves to our evolutionary potential. We reboot the endocrine system. In this way we can restore the balance.

Humans lived for many millions of years this way in the Paleolithic or Stone Age period, and for only a few thousand that humans have grown grain. From an evolutionary standpoint, a diet high in carbohydrate changed the female body in the blink of an eye. That is why your body will quickly accept eating a high-fat low-carbohydrate diet. But you can reach across the chasm of years and decades to change it back. You were born in ketosis and you stayed in ketosis if you were breast fed because breast milk is filled with the fat you needed to develop your nervous system and endocrine system. Breastfed or not (I wasn't), every single one of menopausal symptoms can be remedied by eating fat and very few carbohydrates.

In ketosis you burn fat instead of glucose. Your metabolism switches metabolic tracks. Before their villages became flooded with carbohydrate-heavy foods, the Inuit ate only fat and protein. Researchers marveled they were disease free. Hunter-gatherers who lived in less austere environments were not carbohydrate-driven machines either. They ate a high-fat, low-carbohydrate diet with moderate-protein diet, that was rich in densely packed nutrients taken from berries, herbs and fresh greens. The fat was packed with energy, double the energy coming from protein and carbohydrates. Though our primate ancestors lived on plants, our human brains evolved when we started eating meat and fat.

What is Fat?

Fat comes from different sources, both animal and plant, but it is the animal fat that is more easily synthesized by the body. All the fat we eat is made up of three kinds of fat: saturated, monounsaturated, and polyunsaturated, in different amounts. Butterfat is 31% saturated, 24% unsaturated, and 3% polyunsaturated. Coconut oil is 73.5% saturated fat and 6.5% monounsaturated fat. Lard is pig fat and is 39%, 45% monounsaturated, and 11% polyunsaturated. Animal fats also have varying amounts of eicosapentaenoic acid, EPA and docosahexaenoic acid DHA, the essential omega-3 fatty acids that are involved in various biological functions. Plant oils, such as Flaxseed oil have omega-3 fatty acid in the form of alpha-linolenic acid (ALA) which while it is a fatty acid, is more difficult for humans to convert for use. It is best to get a variety of fats.

The fats to avoid are processed fats and oil, such as margarine and vegetable oil, because the human body cannot metabolize them. Other vegetable oils such as corn and canola oil have also been hydrogenated. The process of hydrogenation keeps them from hardening and makes them impossible to break down. They are not easily burnt as energy and accumulate to cause inflammation. The fact that plastic is made by the same process should make it clear that these oils should not be in your body.

Cholesterol

We eat fat in order to turn it into fatty acids to use as energy. Fat is the best energy we can get. It also gives us the right amount of energy to allow the liver to make cholesterol, which becomes the membrane of every cell in our body, the structure of our central nervous system, and all of our steroid hormones, including vitamin D. Cholesterol is at the top of the hormone cascade, and it takes a lot of energy to synthesize each and every one of those hormones, to end up with estrogen. Fat is not just your fuel—it's your medicine. The energy from the fat you eat will give all your cells energy to restore the ailing physiological functions damaged by high cortisol, inflammation, and high insulin levels. None of this works if you are metabolizing "sugar" of any kind, be it lactose, maltose, sucrose fructose, or glucose. These are present in milk, bread, pasta, honey, carrots, potatoes— even fruit.

Without carbohydrates--which turn into sugars—in your system, you will be eating a higher ratio of fat to protein. This ketogenic state will lower your cortisol levels, improve your resistance to insulin, and reduce inflammation. Inflammation is part of your immune system and how your body protects itself from anything harmful. It could be damaged cells, irritants, pathogens, and even stimuli. Tissue, organs, and cells heat up to burn up what could potentially damage you before healing begins. But constant inflammation, which happens when the level of cortisol stays high, burns you up instead, and causes chronic illness and aging.

Fat and the Brain

The brain needs a huge amount of energy, and it prefers to get this through fat, in the form of ketones. People are taking supplements of DHA and EPA to improve cognitive function, when they could be eating fat. The liver can't make essential fatty acids. Fat only needs three enzymes in the human cell to produce energy. To turn carbohydrate into energy it takes twenty-three. In ketosis, your metabolism becomes direct and simple. There is no smoke. Ketone energy—which is derived from fat—is the cleanest energy for the brain. It increases, recharges, and repairs mitochondria, which are the batteries of your cells. It also protects your neurons from degeneration, which is the cause of such diseases as Alzheimer's and Parkinson's. High cortisol levels cause neurons to burn out, but fat restores them.

Fat and the Adrenals

Just like the liver, the adrenal glands need energy to synthesize steroid hormones. Researchers figured this out in 1988; they were tinkering with estrogen receptors in female rats, trying to find a way to prevent synthetic estrogen from causing tumor growth in breast tissue.[12] Humans are the only primates whose adrenal glands produce steroid hormones along this pathway. It is a pathway completely different from the one the reproductive organs use to produce estrogen and androgen hormones. These researchers invented a new "ology," calling it Intracrinology.[13] This research is very new, but I believe humans evolved this pathway because we started eating fat, which made the human brain so big that our adrenals evolved to synthesize an extra quantity of androgen hormones to help us think and do all the things we've evolved to do.

So what did they conclude, after discovering this amazing new twist to the human endocrine system? They concluded that because estrogen therapy was so very dangerous, they could go one step backward along the hormone cascade and put DHEA, which is produced in the adrenals, in a pill and then market it as DRT (DHEA replacement therapy) to treat menopausal symptoms. Why not just let the adrenals do it?[14] The problem with this is the one I just mentioned—the adrenal glands need a lot of energy to be able to synthesize these hormones. According to Labrie, et al, who researched how beneficial DHEA would be to menopausal women, adrenal deficiency, or the inability of the adrenals to produce enough estrogens, is another component of aging.[15] They don't go back far enough to get to fat. But we will.

Fat Works Fast

Fat works fast. Eating fat can lower your insulin level in fifteen minutes. Not because you've digested and absorbed it that quickly, but because eating stimulates your parasympathetic nervous system, the part of the central nervous system dedicated to rest and digest. Recovery is very important when you're stressed and restoring your adrenal glands. Mental stress becomes physical stress, and vice versa. The same recovery techniques trainers and coaches use to help boost muscle and immune recovery in athletes can also work for us. We want to perform at our optimal levels in our daily lives, and we want to be restored, just as athletes do. If the sympathetic response is heightened, or we're always on alert and in stress mode, switching over to the parasympathetic nervous system will restore the balance, and put us in recovery mode. Deep breathing stimulates the parasympathetic nervous system, because it stimulates the vagus nerve by proximity. The vagus acts as another balancing pole for the nervous system, and is made up of both sympathetic and parasympathetic fibers. The vagus nerve starts in the brain and runs into the esophagus and the diaphragm before passing into the heart and stomach. This means eating calms us down, because, through eating, the vagus nerve is stimulated. High cortisol provokes an adrenalin rush, which can be inhibited by eating. But eating carbohydrates will actually throw gas on the fire, further increasing the adrenalin response from the sympathetic nervous system. Eating fat, however, will stimulate the vagus nerve and switch on the parasympathetic response, at the same time giving much-needed energy to the adrenal glands handling the stress, effectively settling our nerves.

How To Use Fat To Heal

You need more fat to heal. You may have heard about the nutritional ketogenic diet. It is called the low-carbohydrate high-fat diet, or LCHF. To balance and heal your endocrine system you need a *higher*-fat *lower*-carbohydrate diet. You might be asking, "So can I just start eating fat?" Of course you can, but in order for fat to heal you—which requires a full reboot of your system—it has to be your primary energy source. A gradual change is not what is required now. Gradual changes to our diets brought us here in the first place, though these changes did accelerate dangerously in just the last sixty years with the public maligning of fat and the increase in carbohydrate-laden foods. For fat to do its work, you must get rid of all the insulin-raising carbohydrates, sugars, grains, and starches in your diet. Once your endocrine system has regained its balance, then, if you desire, you can gradually add more carbohydrates: the occasional plate of pasta or slice of cake.

It takes about a month for your metabolism to fully adapt to burning fat. You will begin to feel a positive difference after about a week. If you find yourself craving sugar or starches, ask yourself if you really are hungry, if you've eaten enough fat, and if you're under any particular stress. Is it possible you're simply connecting the carbohydrates with comfort?

In the past, I would spend every holiday baking pies and treats—just like my mother did—but I've since adapted my recipes to be low-carb. Now, I make pies with a buttery nut crumble instead of the flaky piecrust I used to roll out so well. I was famous for my biscuits—just like my grandmother—but now I understand that it was the butter that made those biscuits delicious; the flour was just there to hold the butter together. These days, I can spend more time with my kids during the holidays, because I'm no longer stuck in the kitchen. It's a lot faster to make a rich, fatty roast and buttery vegetable than the multiple-course dinners I used to serve.

So how do you start? The first thing to do is to check your kitchen and fridge for anything with carbohydrates and get rid of them. Yes, the cereal comes from grain, which was grown in a field, but how much nutritional value does it really have?

This stuff has to go:

Grains: bread, cereal, corn, rice, crackers, anything made with flour or meal. Grains contain gluten (which can cause intestinal inflammation in many people) and are high in carbohydrates. Corn is also one of the most genetically altered foodstuffs.

Sugar: this category includes honey, corn syrup, and agave syrup, often found in processed food.

Sugary drinks: including fruit juice.

Processed foods: they contain hidden gluten and additives, such as MSG, that provoke adrenal reactions.

Non-dairy milks, such as oat milk, are extremely high in carbohydrates and refined oils. They became popular with the non-dairy, low-fat craze, and many of them are organic, but still not good for you because of the carbohydrate content and the processed polyunsaturated oil they contain.

Artificial sweeteners: these can cause sugar cravings.

Refined oils: refined oils and trans fats, such as sunflower oil and margarine, are hydrogenated and highly inflammatory.

Starches: potatoes and carrots are high in carbohydrates.

This is what you should stock up on:

Fat

There are several different kinds of fat, and the easiest thing to do is to keep it simple. Buy good butter, tallow, duck fat, or lard. You can even learn to make tallow and lard yourself. Of course, grass-fed butter is easier to find in Ireland than it is in Italy, where you'll have better luck finding cheap extra virgin olive oil. Because olive oil doesn't have the quantity of saturated fat animal fat does, it won't be turned into the energy you need it for. You can put it on your salad, but I don't recommend cooking with it. Butter if available almost everywhere. If you are sensitive to the small amount of casein (milk-protein) in the butter you can use ghee. Ghee is far easier to make than tallow. It won't take a lot to give your body the energy it needs, but you will need to consume more than you are likely accustomed to. For the first month, you'll have to add extra fats. After the first month, you should have stabilized your blood sugar enough that you can then get sufficient fat from fatty meats and fish, and from cooking your food in butter and olive oil. However, if your stress level is high, you would do better to continue to eat three times the amount of fat in grams than protein.

Eggs are the perfect food, as they contain equal amounts of fat and protein. Make mayonnaise or keep some boiled eggs ready in the fridge for a quick snack.

Bacon and cheese can have carbohydrates. Look for bacon that has been cured with very little sugar. I suggest using nuts and cheese as snacks. But be aware that some cheeses have more carbohydrates than others. Aged cheeses—such as bleu cheese, Parmesan, and Pecorino—have more fat than fresh cheeses, such as ricotta.

Protein

Protein is regenerative. Animal protein provides all of the essential amino acids necessary for building tissue. It is also the only source of B12 that humans can absorb, and protein provides us with vitamins and minerals. Humans digest protein easily, so there is no waste. There is no indigestible fiber to be eliminated via the colon. However, too much protein *will* go to waste. Just the right amount of protein is used to regenerate connective tissue, but protein leftover from this process will be metabolized as glucose. If you exercise a lot, you will need more protein to rebuild muscle fibers. But remember that too much exercise will also tire your adrenals, so it's best to only exercise gently while your adrenals are healing.

As you transition to a higher-fat lower-carbohydrate diet, I recommend eating simple, unprocessed proteins. This way, it's easier to see how much you're eating and you won't need to read labels. Fatty meats (such as marbled beef and lamb) and fatty fish (such as salmon, anchovies, and bluefish) are rich in Omega 3 fatty acids. Grass-fed meats and wild fish (as opposed to farmed) are also more nutrient dense. As with fat, the protein you consume will really depend on where you live and what is available to you. If you live in the United States, you may have an easier time finding grass-fed beef, which is nearly impossible to obtain in Italy. In Southern Europe, you'll likely be able to procure sardines, anchovies, and lamb.

For health reasons, it's best to eat organic or locally grown foods as much as possible, but depending on where you live, this may be difficult. After all, pollution is everywhere.

Vegetables

Carbohydrates are not essential to life. We know, fat and protein are.[16] Vegetables helped us survive during times when animal protein and fat were scarce. Unfortunately, generations of carbohydrate-heavy diets have made most people insulin resistant and metabolically unhealthy. You can get all your vitamins and minerals from meat. Ruminant animal, such as cows, sheep, deer, and goats eat grass and digest if far better than we can digest vegetables. Their meat is our most nutritious food. Fish is not quite as nutrient dense. It doesn't have as much iron, nor as much fat. Still, all animal protein is more nutritious than vegetables.

It was once believed that vitamin C was the only vitamin not found in meat. The fact that the Inuit people did very well on a high-fat diet without fruit and vegetables confused many doctors following the publication of Vilhjalmur Stefansson's books about the Inuit way of eating.[18] Stefansson returned to the United States hale and hearty, having adopted the "Eskimo-style" diet during his 1908–1918 Arctic expeditions. In 1928, he decided to prove to naysayers that all essential nutrients could be derived from a meat-only diet.[19] In a yearlong study, he and a colleague followed the "Eskimo-style", during which they ate only fatty meat. Eventually, it was discovered that organ meat is particularly rich in vitamin C. A diet high in carbohydrates creates a greater need for vitamin C.

Either way, you can eat leafy green vegetables and still be in ketosis. But you don't have to. Although they contain very few carbohydrates, they are full of anti-nutrients that can interfere with digestion and nutrient absorption. Those with autoimmune conditions may feel better eating just animal foods. If this is too drastic a change for you, stick to leafy greens and asparagus. Some things we think of as vegetables are actually fruit: avocado, beans, pea pods, corn kernels, cucumbers, eggplant, olives peppers, pumpkin, squash, sunflower seeds, red peppers, and tomatoes. They also have more carbohydrates than green leafy vegetables. Grain, nuts, and seeds are also fruit. So stick with green, leafy vegetables until your blood sugar is balanced and your cortisol level is low. Again, what you consume will depend on where you live.

Fruit

Fruit is another nutrient that is not as nutritious than you've been led to think. Modern fruit is full of fructose and has been genetically modified to taste sweeter. Before they were especially modified to be so sweet bananas were unpleasantly fibrous. You don't need this kind of fruit. Meat and vegetables will give you all the vitamins and minerals you need. There are, however, fruits that are less sweet; raspberries and blackberries, for instance, are low in carbohydrates. You can eventually choose to enjoy these with heavy cream.

Snacks

While your metabolism adapts, you will need to eat snacks made up of fat and protein. A breakfast of cereal raises your insulin level and then your cortisol level in response to the raised insulin level. With this kind of breakfast you might also be accustomed to crashing between ten thirty and eleven in the morning. You'll have to retrain your cortisol response. By snacking on a small amount of fat and protein when you would normally crash your body chemistry will relearn its natural rhythm, and after a month or so, a good breakfast of fat and protein will carry you through until lunch.

Getting Started

I've put together a "getting started" meal plan using easy-to-find ingredients, but depending on where you live, some of these items may be difficult to source. For this reason, I've chosen not to include a wide variety of recipes. The goal of this book is to make a high-fat low carbohydrate way of eating right for you, and the simpler the meal plan when you're getting started, the easier it is to follow. Like when learning the piano, you start with something easy —"Chopsticks," for instance—and then when you've learned the basics, you can begin to branch out and try more elaborate songs.

Obviously, we can't always control the food that's placed in front of us. We want to visit friends and family and go to restaurants. I've included tips for these occasions. Many websites and apps can tell you the macronutrient content of a food item, and this can help you substitute ingredients. Unfortunately, most of these sites still count calories, push cardio-based exercise, and try to minimize your fat intake, but remember that isn't the goal. That is what got us here in the first place.

The Basics

What is most important is to understand the basics. The macronutrients— fat and protein, create the foundation. Food is nourishment. It gives us the energy and components our bodies need to function properly. When your blood sugar is balanced, you will feel better, and you won't need to eat foods that are not good for you. Of course, they may be all around you—they may be what your friends are eating. But remember that these kinds of food have been engineered in the comparatively brief period of time following the advent of agriculture. Even though advertisements push them, and many foods seem to define certain cultures (like tomatoes in Italy), we know they are only recent additions to their diet. When you feel better you can consider adding different low-carbohydrate vegetables, one at a time. They aren't necessary for nutrition—your getting all you need from animal foods. Think of them as entertainment.

Eat lots of good fat. How do you know how much fat you need to consume? First, weigh yourself. Once your insulin and cortisol levels are stabilized, any excess weight will come off. Often, insulin resistance causes water retention, because the inflammation is so high. Remember, what is important is how you feel, and not the numbers you see on the scale.

I would suggest weighing yourself in kilograms. The number of kilograms you weigh is the same number of grams of net protein you will need per day. This is for an average activity level. However, if you're training for a marathon or work out more than three times a week, you will need more protein to regenerate tissues. How much you exercise is also an important aspect of lowering cortisol and reducing insulin resistance, but I will discuss that later in this chapter.

As an example, if you weigh 60 kilograms, you will need 100 grams of net protein a day. Or, if you're measuring in imperial, if you weigh 130 pounds, you will need 100 grams of protein a day. This is a moderate protein diet, because right now, you should be concentrating on the amount of fat you're eating. Both protein and fat are filling, which means that if you eat too much protein, you won't be able to eat enough fat. Protein in excess will also be metabolized as glucose. Fat will never be burned as glucose, only as ketones. While protein *is* important, it doesn't have fat's anti-inflammatory effect.

Now that you have calculated how much protein you need to eat, you can easily figure out how much fat you'll need eating one half more grams fat than protein. So if you're eating 100 grams of protein, you will need at least 150 grams of fat each day for the first month. (Of course, I'm rounding these numbers. A few grams more or less isn't important; focus instead on the ratio of fat to protein). The fat to protein ratio looks like 80% fat and 20% protein. This will likely be more fat than you're used to eating. You've probably been led to think that eating fat will make you fat, that it will accumulate as cholesterol, and that this will give you heart disease. None of this is true.[20]

Numerous studies, such as the Framingham Heart Study, have tried to link cholesterol to heart disease, but they have found no link. A little bit of digging into the researchers and doctors promoting the use of statins (cholesterol-lowering medications) uncovers a story almost exactly like the one about synthetic and conjugated estrogens. The fact remains that people who do not take statins and eat high amounts of fat and very little carbohydrate have lower cholesterol levels. Studies of women in Japan who have higher LDL cholesterol—the supposedly "bad" cholesterol—showed that they had lower breast cancer rates, suggesting that LDL, a protein that carries cholesterol to various parts of the body that need it, was actually protective.[21] This confounded Western researchers just as much as the Inuit Paradox, and soon researchers were theorizing that the phytoestrogens, such as soy, were the real protective element in their diet.[22] But as of 2014, the rate of cholesterol in Japan is still on the rise, while the rate of coronary heart disease is still going down. What is protecting the Japanese from heart disease? Animal fat.

Without glucose in your system, you'll burn fat instead, which means that fat won't accumulate as adipose tissue or as arterial plaque. If you have high inflammation, or an autoimmune condition such as Hashimoto's Thyroiditis, you may have high cholesterol levels, but this is not because of the fat you eat. Cholesterol protects from heart disease. Low-fat diets increase insulin resistance and lower how much fat you burn. Those egg-white omelets with a side of toast are what create inflammation, not that egg yolk.

"Getting Started" Good Fat Meal Plan

This is an example of a daily higher-fat lower-carb meal plan if you weigh 60 kg or 132 lbs.

Breakfast

2 eggs fried in 1–2 tbsp butter with 3 pieces of bacon.

or

1 egg scrambled in butter with 50 g smoked salmon.

or

Butterccino

It's important to have a blender to make this into a 'ccino. The blender froths the butter to a nice foamy consistency. You can just stir in the butter, but it isn't the same. I've just stirred it in while traveling, because the butter is my fuel. If you really want to improve adrenal function, I do recommend eventually weaning off of coffee and drinking decaffeinated coffee only.

1 cup of brewed coffee whipped with

2 tbsp (25 g) butter

If you are not hungry or you find it difficult to eat breakfast:

Eggoccino

1 cup of brewed coffee whipped with

2 tbsp (25 g) butter

1 raw egg

These breakfasts will give you enough protein and enough fat to energize you and dampen the cortisol fire.

Snack

If your adrenals have been pumping out a lot of cortisol, you'll usually experience a dip in energy around 11 a.m. This is why a mid-morning snack is important.

The snack should provide both fat and protein.

Cheese, like eggs, contains half fat and half protein. Some cheeses are higher in fat, like gorgonzola and cream cheese. But aged cheeses—pecorino, cheddar and parmesan, have the most fat and the least sugar—lactose. Goat and sheep's milk cheeses are made from A2 milk which some people may find easier to digest

Cured meats, such as prosciutto, have both protein and fat. However, you'll want to avoid lean meats. When it comes to smoked and cured meats, bear in mind that today the smoking and curing process does involve additives to which some people are sensitive. The more inflammation in your system, the more sensitive you will be to additives. If you live in a city, you will likely be able to find high-quality cured meats. Always read the labels, and choose the product with the fewest additives.

Or, keep it simple: eat a piece of butter with a piece of cheese.

1 oz (30 g) high-fat cheese with 1 tbsp butter. You can use the cheese as a plate. Eat them together. This is fuel for your adrenals. You can also wrap it up in a piece of lettuce or arugula.

or

1 oz (30g) high-fat cured meat with 1 tbsp butter

or

1 oz of any fresh or dried high-fat meat or fish with 1 tbsp butter

Drink a large glass of water with your snack.

Lunch

If you weren't hungry at breakfast, you will likely be hungry now.

Depending upon your stress levels, the eggoccino coffee with butter you had for breakfast should sustain you for about four hours.

5 oz (150 g) protein with 2 tbsp butter. This can be any kind of fresh meat, fish, or an egg preparation (such as an

omelet or a frittata). A can of sardines or tuna in olive oil is also a simple lunch protein. Just make sure you either cook it in fat or add fat to it after it is cooked. The butter, or any other fat you choose, is crucial to get you up to that 80:20 ratio of fat to protein to quickly switch your metabolism from glycolytic to ketotic. The French love plopping a piece of fresh butter on their entrecôte.

If you eat at work, you can get a sandwich and skip the bread. If you're eating your sandwich on the run, use the bread as a vessel for the protein—just don't eat the bread. Mayonnaise is also a good way to add more fat to your lunch.

Afternoon Snack

This snack is designed to keep your blood sugar and cortisol levels stable throughout the afternoon. For many people, the afternoon is the hardest part of the day. Stress tends to culminate around three o'clock, which is why the Germans have their coffee and cake at this hour, the British their tea and sandwiches, the Italians their merenda, and so on. The reason these afternoon pick-me-ups are made of glucose with some caffeine or nicotine to wash it down is because these stimulate the adrenals, which raises cortisol and will make you crave sugar or alcohol. Biochemically they are the same thing. Unfortunately, you soon find you need something stronger, and often this is met with things like the aperitivo in Italy and happy hour in the United States.

If you like to drink coffee at this hour, make it a decaffeinated butterccino (the same as from breakfast), but skip the egg. Decaffeinated butter coffee is a great way to ensure you're getting enough fat during the day, and sometimes it's a challenge to get the therapeutic amount of fat to calm cortisol sensitivity.

1 oz (30 g) high-fat cheese with 1 tbsp butter

or

1 oz (30 g) high-fat cured meat with 1 tbsp butter

or

1 oz of any fresh or dried high-fat meat or fish with 1tbsp butter

Drink a large glass of water with your snack.

Dinner

The macronutrients for dinner are the same as for lunch. You can have your protein cooked any way you like, so long as it is cooked or roasted in butter, tallow, or lard.

If you like, you can have a glass of wine with dinner. You will be in ketosis after two days, and when you're in ketosis, you'll be more sensitive to alcohol. Remember, your liver is now your energy factory—it's the liver that turns the fat into fatty acids and then ketone energy. Wine has sugar alcohols and not too many carbohydrates. Beer, however, is basically bread in a glass, filled with gluten and carbohydrates, and should be avoided.

How to Know if You Are in Ketosis

It will take a couple of days to get the glucose out of your system. Ketosis will let you know if you are eating enough fat so that you can burn fat instead of glucose. You can check this by measuring your ketones with Ketostix, which can be obtained inexpensively at the pharmacy or online. The instructions tell you to pee into a container and then dip the Ketostix into your urine (or you can just pee on the stick). The Ketostixs will measure excess ketones, meaning the ones produced by your liver, but not used for energy. If you burnt them through exercise or activity you won't have any leftover to measure. For this reason, it's best to do this test after you have eaten.

Don't worry too much if the stick doesn't turn pink or purple. Some people naturally produce very few ketones, and a particularly stressful day will force some glucose into your system. There will always be some glucose; after all, the liver produces it during the night to fuel your brain as you sleep. You simply don't want to burn glucose as your main form of energy. At first check to see if you're in ketosis at various times of the day. If you find a particular time of day when the ketones show up on the Ketostix, keep checking at that time, and make note of what you ate until that time, so you can know what works. For instance, if you eat a breakfast with a lot of fat, you will have some extra ketones before you go about your day and burn them. There are three types of ketones: beta-hydroxybutyrate, acetoacetate, and acetone. The Ketostix can only measure acetoacetate, and there is usually only excess acetoacetate during the first month while your metabolism is adapting to burning fat. In the end, this is about how you feel, not how many ketones you have left over.

Going Out for Meals

Most restaurants offer protein and fat options. Pizzerias, for instance, also serve cold cuts and anchovies. Mexican restaurants usually serve dishes with avocado (such as guacamole) and seared beef. Even if you can only find protein-only dishes, simply eat a piece of cheese with butter or a boiled egg before going to the restaurant. Coffee places usually have pats of butter, so don't be shy: plop the butter into your coffee. Dare to be different!

While restaurants have set menus, you can usually get creative with your choices as long as you don't ask them to cook something special for you. You can't remove ingredients from sauces, but you *can* ask the server to take away the bread. However, bear in mind that sometimes merely asking for something different can offend an establishment. Often they're so used to serving their dishes in one particular way or they believe theirs is the way a dish "ought" to be served. Some people are afraid of change, so don't take their offense personally. When you go out your friends and family may also challenge your new way of eating or insist that it's bad for you. Fortunately, once they see how much better you're feeling, they will usually shut up. Alternately, they might begin feeling insecure and defensive about their own diet and bring up articles they read that contradict you. Food shaming is nothing new. Simply remember that the facts have always been twisted to serve certain interests and that you are in charge of your own health.

How Are You Going to Feel These Changes?

It will only take twenty-four hours to change your metabolism, for your body to burn through all the glucose and start burning fat. But it may take longer for your body to adapt to burning fat instead of glucose for energy. It may take a few days for your biochemistry to adjust. Healing is not linear; it may come in waves, so you may notice a few days of big changes followed by hardly anything at all. But that doesn't mean nothing is happening inside your body. Healing works from the top down and the inside out.

This Is What You Can Expect to Experience Right Away

You will lose the water your body retained in order to keep cool while it labored through the twenty-three enzymatic processes involved in creating one molecule of energy from glucose. This water has been stored in your tissues—sometimes in your ankles, upper arms, thighs, or around the belly. You will lose this water through urination.

You'll find your energy level will increase as soon as you start burning fat. If it doesn't, that means your metabolism hasn't fully adapted yet. If your energy level still hasn't improved after a month, you should check your thyroid function. Some underlying conditions may reveal themselves after the mask of glucose has been removed. The breakfast mentioned earlier in this section will give you longer-lasting energy, which means you won't need that mid-morning pick-me-up in the form of a coffee (caffeine), a cigarette (nicotine), or a pastry (refined sugar and flour).

It typically takes about a week for hot flashes to subside, depending on your cortisol rhythm and how irregular it is. In most cases, morning and evening hot flashes will become less intense. The night sweats will disappear, and you'll wake up less frequently during the night. Because your body and mind will no longer go automatically into stress-mode, your cortisol levels will stabilize, and your body will not react by having a hot flash. However, it may take some time for them to go away completely. After all, your body remembers how it used to get your attention. If you're extra tired, or if you eat something that doesn't agree with you, you may have an inflammatory reaction. Fortunately, it will be easier to recognize the cause of this response and avoid triggering it in future.

Your moods will also become more even. Your lows won't go so far down, and yes, your highs will be less high —but remember, it's dangerous to fly too high. In the moment, it may feel good to breathe the ether, but it *is* a stress and coming down is still a crash. Your serotonin and dopamine levels will stabilize and will more easily transmit those feelings of happiness, initiative, and optimism.

Your muscles and joints will stop aching. With less inflammation, that pain in your hip, elbow, shoulder, or neck that usually flares up when you are tired or stressed will no longer do that to get your attention. As mentioned earlier, this may come back when you're tired, but that's normal.

You will digest better. Our bodies aren't really equipped to digest grain. It causes inflammation, causing both Candida bacteria to take over your gut and the valves on either end of your intestines (the pyloric valve, which leads from the stomach to the small intestine, and the ileocecal valve, which separates the small intestine from the large intestine) to become inflamed. This can cause leaky gut syndrome, which involves irritable bowel syndrome, bloating, gas, and abdominal pain. When your cortisol levels are lower, the gallbladder is more easily stimulated to secrete the important bile acids that digest your food.

Your mind will be clearer. Fat is essential for your brain to function, and it's also the only way to synthesize vitamin D. The gallbladder digests fat, and if you've been avoiding fat for much of your life, your gallbladder may have stopped functioning properly. One of the problems with the low-fat diet is that it can cause gallstones. The bile acids sit unused in the gallbladder and over time become hard and dense. Many of my patients in their seventies have had their gallbladders removed, and this can cause memory problems.

Orgasms will be easier to achieve and more pleasurable. By reducing your cortisol level, your body will find it easier to relax. The parasympathetic system controls rest, digestion, and the ability to stimulation as well as vaginal lubrication and erection. The clitoris is essentially a tiny penis, and it also becomes erect when stimulated.

You will sleep better. When your cortisol rhythm is stable, you won't lie awake in the dark, fidgeting. Your muscles won't cramp or spasm. You won't wake up at four in the morning to pee. Though you may still wake up once in the night, you'll go back to sleep more easily and your sleep will be deeper.

With low vitamin D, your bones will be brittle. With high cortisol, you'll also have brittle bones. Vitamin D comes from fat; you can lie out in the sun all you want, but it takes both sun and fat to synthesize vitamin D. There isn't a lot of sun where the Inuit live, but their diet of fatty fish and organ meat provided them with the fat-soluble vitamins A and D for strong bones. What did European sailors, suffering from rickets and scurvy, eat on their long voyages? Biscuits. How much fat do you suppose Tiny Tim, from Charles Dickens's *A Christmas Carol,* had in his diet? Did he eat enough protein?[23] London skies were clouded with soot, which interfered with UV-B rays and vitamin D absorption, and the poor mostly ate bread. Dickens himself wrote, "One of the worst forms of scrofula—rachitism, or rickets . . . arises under the influence of chilly dwellings an insufficient alimentation [nourishment] . . . and milk deprivation in infants."[24]

Collagen makes hair lustrous and skin soft and elastic. You can, of course, get collagen from expensive conditioners and skin creams, but these will never work as well as the collagen you eat. These creams are also full of chemical xenoestrogens, which disrupt the endocrine system. If you're not digesting fat, collagen will turn into fibroids in adipose tissue.[25] Androgen hormones—both estrogen and testosterone—influence skin quality and promote the healing of wounds because they increase collagen deposition.[26] But why rub a synthetic hormone on your skin? Eating and metabolizing fat means you will produce the amount of hormones to keep your hair full and shiny and your skin smooth and elastic. If skin aging is due to inflammation and oxidation, you can reduce both by eating fat.

The same goes for your breasts. They need fat too. While excess estrogen (either produced in reaction to high insulin levels or from synthetic hormones) can make your breasts swell and feel tender and lumpy, fat gives them fullness. It won't happen overnight, but your breasts will regain what they lost when your body thought it was starving. Eating and metabolizing fat won't suddenly give you big breasts, but it will restore fat to where it is supposed to be, as a hormonal reserve.

Not all women like this. Many women feel uncomfortable with their bodies, and especially in adolescence, breasts often bring unwanted attention. For most women, it is the first time they feel objectified. I certainly did; I'm sure that one of the reasons I started dieting was to get rid of my breasts. Then, after nursing three children, I complained that my breasts looked like two empty Ziploc bags. Did I eat fat? No. I also ran fifty miles every week. (As I've said, I made all the mistakes I'm now advising you against.) After a year of eating fat I didn't gain weight; my breasts breasts returned to how they were before I had kids, so that while they didn't get bigger, they got fuller. I have to admit it took some getting used to. Women have two primary places their bodies store fat: the breasts and the buttocks. You don't need plastic surgery to restore your breasts.

If you think you're overweight, make sure you're not comparing yourself to someone who is very thin. Our bodies come in all shapes and sizes, and unfortunately, the clothing industry has created an obsession with cookie-cutter bodies that are almost impossible to realize with a healthy endocrine system. Know that what is considered good-looking in our current times is not necessarily what your body is designed for. In Ancient Greece and Rome, for instance, the unibrow was all the rage. Women used to attach dyed goat hair to their foreheads with tree resin to get the right look!

Where does beauty come from? Is someone trying to sell you a style or a shape? We know body fat is essential for survival. Is it beautiful if it isn't working? Fat is a vitally important endocrine organ. It has a job to do. It makes hormones, which improve insulin sensitivity, regulate body temperature, maintain muscle tissue, and reduce inflammation.[27] Insulin is supposed to move fat in and out of cells on a continual basis as needed for energy, but if there's insulin resistance, fat cells become blocked and triglycerides get stuck inside them. When this happens, adipose tissue no longer moves through the system but accumulates around organs, such as the liver and the heart. Insulin resistance turns circulating fat into fibrotic tissue in the uterus and breasts. But we need to maintain the right amount of body fat, not whittle it away. Recommendations for body mass index (BMI) have been lowered in synchrony with cholesterol levels. Each time recommendations for cholesterol levels have been lowered by medical guidelines, so have the BMI. Thin women have fertility issues. The risk of Ovulatory Disorder is increased for women with a BMI below 20.[28] The rate of nonalcoholic fatty liver disease is reaching epidemic proportions in women, with studies showing that it occurs in women with either very low or very high BMI.[29] Non-alcoholic fatty liver disease (NAFLD) is also related to polycystic ovary syndrome (PCOS), which is caused by insulin resistance.[30] Fat is not bad—insulin resistance is.

The problem is that what most women want is to be is thin. Low-calorie diets and overtraining wreak havoc on the endocrine system. Your body is programmed to have some fat on it. The right amount of dietary fat will take stress off the liver; too little will force the liver to produce more cholesterol. High insulin and cortisol levels lock lipids into cells, keeping them out of circulation. When we think of the word "malnourished," we tend to picture someone who is emaciated, but for someone with fatty liver disease, it is the fact that their bodies cannot burn fat because it only burns carbohydrates and the fat accumulates in the liver. Obesity is also a form of malnourishment caused by the wrong kind of nourishment, which is too many carbohydrates. If someone is too thin, overtrained, or simply not consuming enough fat, their pancreas will have to produce more insulin to protect the vital organs and build fat around them to ensure they get energy.

You'll also have more energy with which to exercise. Don't over-exercise, or run yourself and your body into the ground. If you exercise too much, it will no longer be fun, but stressful. It's good to move. Moving circulates blood and lymph, eliminating toxins, and it shuttles oxygen and nutrients all around your body. Your muscles protect your bones and joints, and they store oxygen, energy, and hormones. They need fat in order to move smoothly. A high-fat, low-carbohydrate diet will give you the energy you need to exercise. Amino acids and collagen from animal protein will provide plenty of raw material for muscle and skin growth.

Exercise that requires you to increase your heart rate for longer than twenty-five minutes will make your cortisol levels go up. It tricks your body into thinking you're actually running away from something—not just putting in the miles on a treadmill. Medical guidelines always emphasize diet and exercise. But that is what got us here. It may work for a while when you are younger, but after too much diet and exercise your endocrine system puts a stop to it. That's why it no longer works.

During the first month, activities such as hiking, walking, or gentle concentrated movement, such as Taiji, will benefit you more than intense exercises where trainers often say to do it until you "feel the burn in your muscles." If you are feeling the burn, it's because you are on fire, and there is inflammation.

What Else Can Happen?

Most women will feel good after just these changes. Depending upon such things as your stress levels, how many years you've been on the pill, and how frequently you pushed yourself putting in those miles, your body chemistry may be more or less cranky. It depends on the tilt of your wobble: more tilt and it will take your body more energy to regain balance.

You May Need More Salt

Carbohydrates cause your body to retain water and salt; this is because of all the work your metabolism has to do to turn glucose into energy. You lose salt and water in the first week of ketosis, which means you will need to make sure to replenish these. Make sure you drink one and a half to two liters of water a day. Salting your food with an unprocessed, natural salt (such as Himalayan salt), will give you not only sodium, but also important trace minerals that are harder to get from other sources. The iodine in processed iodized salt actually evaporates as soon as you open the container. It is better to eat a small amount of seaweed or sprinkle natural kelp powder along with good salt on your food for your iodine needs. Salting your regular meals will easily give you a teaspoon of Himalayan salt a day. Salt does not make you retain water, carbohydrates do.

Other Minerals

Since a diet high in carbohydrates robs your body of nutrients, including minerals, switching to a high-fat diet means you will have to wake up all the receptors that have become accustomed to making do with less than what they need. Your body needs to be reminded that you are changing your energy source. Your adrenals need magnesium to turn fat into hormones and also in order to rest after having worked so hard for you. You can get enough magnesium from your food, but when you first make the switch, you may experience cramps in your muscles, which means you have a deficiency and will need to take supplements. Usually 500 milligrams of magnesium glycinate, which is the more bioavailable kind, taken nightly, is enough.

Changing the Digestive Demographic

It takes certain enzymes and bacteria to digest carbohydrates. The bacteria that break down carbohydrates are different from those that eat and transform protein and fat. Although there are enzymes in your saliva that start the process of metabolizing your food, crucial substances for breaking down fat and protein, have to be abundant in your stomach and small intestine. If you've been primarily eating carbohydrates (this includes vegetables) for some time, you will need to increase the hydrochloric acid, bile, lipase and protease needed to break down protein and fat. These digestive aids may have become reduced on a high-carbohydrate diet. Furthermore, stress reduces the quantity of both all of these substances. The bacteria that live on carbohydrates are different from the one that live on meat and fat. I haven't found any sold as supplements, but rest assured—the microbiome changes completely, from carbohydrate-eating bacteria to meat-eating bacteria, in up to two weeks. Supplementing initially with betaine-HCL, bile salts, lipase , and protease until your reserve increases will ensure that you can absorb all of the nutrients from your food, and that the transition from carbohydrates to fat and protein goes smoothly. As the glucose-loving bacteria die off, you may for a few days experience some gas.

Take Care of Your Liver

You should always take care of your liver. The liver is where old hormones go to be recycled. Excess estrogen is sometimes stored in the liver on a high-carbohydrate diet. Toxins also go to the liver to be eliminated. Not only does your liver produce bile, which is essential for breaking down fat into molecules for digestion, but the fatty acids from that process go back into your liver, where they are turned into ketones. This is what you'll be burning if you do not eat glucose. This means fat will be turned into energy. If you don't burn fat, it will accumulate in your liver—also known as fatty liver disease. Fructose and alcohol are the worst offenders, because they go directly to the liver, where most of it is turned into fat. Your liver is busy making energy. Just by removing high-carbohydrate foods that turn into the glucose and fructose that clog the liver, you will be taking care of your liver.

Cravings

Usually if you eat enough fat, you won't have any cravings. After a couple of days, you'll be naturally hungry when you need food.

Circadian Rhythm

If you're sensitive to cortisol—which you may be, depending upon your stress level—you will have to be patient with your endocrine system. It may be somewhat over-reactive. Remember that you're taking better care of yourself than you have for a long time, and if you've been ignoring your body's warnings, it may have taken to yelling at you. For instance, waking up in the middle of the night with a pounding heart doesn't usually mean there's something wrong with your heart; rather, it means you're having an adrenalin reaction. Your adrenals may think they have to start waking you at four in the morning so that you get up in time for work, instead of gently waking you at seven.

The hormones cortisol and melatonin respond to light and dark. Our bodies have evolved to be awake and to look for food, eat, and work during the day, and to sleep and restore during the night. Of course, you can force your body to stay awake longer. Many people have to spend some portion of their lives working the night shift. While dancing all night may be fun once in a while, working the night shift is hard on the endocrine system because it disrupts the circadian rhythm. This is another example of pulling on one strand of the endocrine web. Parents of newborns know how hard it is to wake up several times during the night. When you stay up late you tend to wake up at the same time in the morning. This is because your adrenals start secreting cortisol at around 4 a.m. Production rises fairly gradually until 9 a.m. and then starts to decline very gently until 6 p.m., when most people are either still at work or just leaving the office. This is where happy hour comes in; your body is telling you that it's time go home and rest, but by the time you finish work, get home, and maybe run some errands, you won't be able to have dinner until around eight or nine. Happy hour, or an aperitivo, will keep you going until you can actually sit down to dinner.

For most people, by the time you want to lie down in bed and go to sleep, you have completely confused your adrenals by pushing your body past the time when it needs dinner. You might have done this by having a drink (alcohol stimulates the adrenals) or by going to the gym, because the evening is the only time you can get there. So now your circadian rhythm is off-kilter. Melatonin, produced by the pineal gland and which puts you to sleep, should have been pumping gently from 6 p.m. on, but instead you've forced your adrenals to pump out cortisol to allow you to stay awake. That's why you wake up in the middle of the night to go to the bathroom—not because you can't hold it, but because this (and through nightmares and palpitations) is one of the only ways your adrenals can communicate with you. They're trying to take care of you. If you do wake up, eat a piece of cheese or butter to help lower the cortisol response and get you back to sleep.

Babies don't have this problem. They just fall asleep when they're tired or stressed. They conk out in your arms, in the stroller, or wherever they are, and just switch off. As adults, we have forgotten how to do that. You just need to turn off all the alarms by eating fat, and you will relearn how. The endocrine system operates on a twenty-eight-day cycle (for men too), and this is why it takes about a month for your metabolism to adapt to burning fat. The first step to righting any imbalances in your endocrine system is to eat a high-fat, low-carbohydrate diet. After a month, you can begin to add more variety to your diet. You may want to eat more protein or some low-sugar fruit, such as berries. You can experiment with foods that are lower in carbs, but always keep in mind you may be sensitive to anti-nutrients in some vegetables.

Many of my patients return to the higher fat/lower carbohydrate diet because it makes them feel better. They may add more vegetables or more meat, or they'll eat fewer vegetables and just add fat to their morning coffee. They might come back to it after a particularly stressful time, with work or family, or both. Some use it as a way to get back on track after traveling and eating different foods. As I said before, I have changed a lot of the dishes I cook at holidays, but sometimes I make them the same way I did when I cooked with flour and sugar. It only takes one day of going back to the higher fat/lower carb meal plan get back into ketosis.

Everyone is different, but everyone has to eat the right amount of fat for their energy needs, and large amounts of carbohydrates and sugar will never be good for the body. If you are ill or recovering, you need fat to get better. Because it is anti-inflammatory and protects the nervous system, a high-fat diet maintains the body's balance in times of stress. Once you are well, you only need fat to burn as fuel. Your liver will make all the cholesterol you need. Choosing fatty foods—such as skirt steaks, pork chops, wild salmon and mackerel, fish, eggs, and maybe avocados, adding more fats such as butter, tallow, and lard—can often provide enough fat to give you the energy you need. You'll see, and you'll learn what works for you based on how you feel.

What kind of woman do you want to be?

Society prepares little girls for adolescence and the trials of pain and discomfort that are supposed to come with it. Women are prepared in the same way for menopause, and now peri-menopause. As little girls we are just children; we have the same illnesses that our brothers have. With puberty, we are separated from "humans" in general and become "women." Somehow, our bodies are no longer good enough. Young men aren't offered hormones, but young women who don't menstruate at a certain age are taken to the gynecologist and prescribed hormones. If she bleeds too much, she is again given hormones. She's prescribed hormones to make sure she doesn't get pregnant and prescribed them if she cannot. Then, as soon as her periods become irregular again, she is given more hormones. If she gives birth and hemorrhages, they take out her ovaries. Of course, without her ovaries she will be prescribed more hormones. They vary in quantity—more estrogen here, a little progesterone there. Perhaps with an antidepressant to take the edge off, and now that she's finally menopausal, they can add in some estrogen receptors or selective estrogen receptor modulators (SERM) to prevent osteoporosis.

This chaos started with an endocrine imbalance. Estradiol (E2)is the absolute last steroid hormone produced on the hormone cascade. Fat, or cholesterol, goes in seven different directions before becoming estradiol, and that's the simplest route, the one without any problems. Why hasn't anyone looked at the other possible causes of endocrine imbalance? Because, well, because it was assumed that a woman's body was made exclusively for procreation, so if there's anything wrong, that's how you fix it.

But now you know this isn't true. You were born a woman, and that means you have the organs and the hormones to bear children. Evolution has given you the option.

Whether you choose to have children or not is entirely up to you. Menstruation was never intended to bring pain and discomfort, just as menopause was not supposed to come with symptoms. Menopause is just as the word itself signifies: an end to menstruation. How can you make this a great time of your life? Eat a mostly (or all) animal based diet with lots of fat, some protein, and very few carbohydrates. You and your menopause will be amazing.

References

Preface

National Women's Health Network, *Hysterectomy in the United States: Background, 2015*, https://www.nwhn.org/hysterectomy/, accessed December 28, 2018.

Tyson, M.D., Andrews, P. E., Ferrigni, R. F., Humphreys, M. R., Parker, A. S., & Castle, E. P. (2016). *Radical Prostatectomy Trends in the United States: 1998 to 2011*, Mayo Clinic Proceedings, 91(1), p.10

Ornella Moscucci, *The Science of Woman: Gynaecology andgender in England, 1800-1929*, Cambridge University Press, 1990, p. 2

World Health Organization, *The Global Burden of Chronic*, https://www.who.int/nutrition/topics/2_background/en/ , accessed December 28, 2018.

Introduction

1. E. F. Angell Drake, *What a Woman of Forty-Five Ought to Know*, Self and Sex Series, The Vir Publishing Company, Philadelphia 1902, p. 30, p. 53, p. 130.

2. M.P. Jacobi, *A Pathfinder in Medicine*, Women's Medical Assn. of New York City, New York 1925, p. 482.

3. J.M. Strange, *In Full Possession of Her Powers: Researching and Rethinking Menopause in early Twentieth-century England and Scotland*, «Society for the Social History of Medicine» Oxford University Press, 2012, p. 694

4. M. Lock, Introduction to *Encounters with Aging: Mythologies of Menopause in Japan and North America*, University of California Press, Berkley 1993, p. xix.

5. L. Gannon, *Women in Health Portraits of Menopause in the Mass Media*, «Women & Health», vol. 27, n. 3, 1998, pp. 1-15.

6. E. Novak, *The Management of the Menopause*, «American Journal of Obstetrics and Gynecology», vol. 40, n. 4, 1940, p. 589.

7. S. E. Bell, *Premenstrual Syndrome and the Medicalization of Menopause: A Sociological Perspective*, in AA.VV. *Premenstrual Syndrome*, Springer, Boston 1987, p.152.

8. G. Zhao, *Menopausal Symptoms: Experience of Chinese Women*, «Climacteric», vol. 3, n. 2, 2000, p. 143.

9. S. E. Bell, *Premenstrual Syndrome and the Medicalization of Menopause: A Sociological Perspective*, in AA.VV. *Premenstrual Syndrome*, Springer, Boston 1987,p 159

10. E. Drake, *What a Woman of Forty-Five Ought to Know*, 1902, p. 30, p. 53, p. 130.

11. N. Collins, *The Real MacLaine* «Vanity Fair», March 1991, p. 144.

Chapter One

What's in a word

1. B. Gardenour, *Gender In Medicine and Natural History*, in AA.VV., *Medieval Science, Technology, and Medicine, An Encyclopedia*, Routledge, New York 2005, pp.182-183.

2. B. Rowland, *Medieval Woman's Guide to Health: The First Gynecological Handbook*, Kent State Press, Kent 1981, p. 61.

3. L. Townsend, *Obstetrics Through the Ages*, «The Medical Journal of Australia», vol.1, n.17, 1952, p. 558-565.

4. G. Savage, *On the Mental Diseases of the Climacteric* (delivered at the Medical Graduates' College and Polyclinic on March 12, 1903), «The Lancet», vol. 162, n. 4183, 1903, p.1209

5. T. Schlich, *Controlled Intervention: The History of Modern Surgery, 1800-1914,*

6. A. Bashford, *Purity and Pollution: Gender, Embodiment and Victorian Medicine,* Spinger, New York 1998, p. 121.

7. M. R. Melendy, *Perfect Womanhood for Maidens-Wives-Brothers*, Monarch Book Co., Chicago 1903, p. 171.

8. B. Seaman, *The Greatest Experiment Ever Performed on Women: Exploding The Estrogen Myth*, Seven Stories Press, New York 2004, p. 13.

9. R. Formanek, *Premodern Views of the Menopause*, in AA.VV. *The Meanings of Menopause*, The Analytic Press, Hillsdale 1990, p. 20.

10. E. Allen, *Ovarian Hormones and Female Genital Cancer*, «Journal of American Medicine», vol. 114, n. 21, 1940,

11. M. A. Shampo, *Adolf Butenandt—Nobel Prize for Chemistry*, «Mayo Clin. Proc», vol. 87, n. 4, 2012, p. 27.

12. B. Seaman, *The Greatest Experiment Ever Performed on Women: Exploding The Estrogen Myth*, Seven Stories Press, New York 2004, p. 28.

13. N. Langston, *Toxic Bodies: Hormone Disruptors and the Legacy of DES*, Yale University Press, New Haven 2011. p.112

14. B. Seaman, *The Greatest Experiment Ever Performed on Women: Exploding The Estrogen Myth*, Seven Stories Press, New York 2004, p. 41.

15. *ibidem*.

16. E. Siegal Watkins, *The Estrogen Elixir: A History of Hormone Replacement Therapy in America*, Johns Hopkins University Press, Baltimore 2007, p. 32.

17. E. Novak, *The Management of The Menopause*, «American Journal of Obstetrics and Gynecology», vol. 40, n. 4, 1940, p.590.

18. E. Siegal Watkins, *The Estrogen Elixir: A History of Hormone Replacement Therapy in America*, Johns Hopkins University Press, Baltimore 2007, p. 34.

19. O. Moscucci, *Cancer in Britain, 1860-1910: The Emergence of Cancer as a Public Health Concern*, «American Journal of Public Health», vol. 95, n.8, 2005, p.1312

20. J.P. Pratt, *The Treatment of Menopause, Southern Medical Journal* 31, 562.

21. E. Novak, *The Management of the Menopause*, American Journal of Obstetrics and Gynocology 1940, 40, p.592

22. R. R. Newbold, *Toxic Bodies: Hormone Disruptors and the Legacy of DES*, «Environmental Health Perspectives» vol. 118, n. 10, 2010, p. 452.

23. *ibidem*.

24. H. Harris, *A Critical View of Three Psychoanalytical Positions on Menopause*, in AA.VV. *The Meanings of Menopause*, The Analytic Press, Hillsdale 1990, p. 65.

25. J. Delaney - M.J. Lupton - E. Toth, *The Curse: A Cultural History of Menstruation*, University of Illinois Press, Chicago 1988, p. 220.

26. T. Benedek, *Psychoanalytic investigations: Selected Papers*, Quandrangle, New York 1973, pp. 322-349.

27. H. J. Eysenck, *The Effects of Psychotherapy: An Evaluation*, «Journal of Consulting Psychology», vol. 16, n. 5, 1952, p.323.

28. L. S. Mitteness, *Historical Changes in Public Information about the Menopause*, «Urban Anthropology», vol. 12, n. 2, 1983, p.161-179.

29. B. Seaman, *The Greatest Experiment Ever Performed on Women: Exploding The Estrogen Myth*, Seven Stories Press, New York 2004, p. 66.

30. E. Siegal Watkins, *The Estrogen Elixir: A History of Hormone Replacement Therapy in America*, Johns Hopkins University Press, Baltimore 2007, p. 64.

31. D. Reuben, *Everything You Ever Wanted to Know About Sex, But Were Afraid To Ask*, David McKay Publications, Philadelphia 1969, p. 283

32. B. Seaman, *The Greatest Experiment Ever Performed on Women: Exploding The Estrogen Myth*, Seven Stories Press, New York 2004, p. 60.

33. *ivi.* p. 50

34 G. Feldberg - M. Ladd-Taylor - A. Li - K. McPherson, a cura di, *Women, Health, and Nation: Canada and the United States Since 1945*, McGill University Press, Montreal 2003, p. 101.

35. Wulf H. Utian, Wikipedia https://en.wikipedia.org/wiki/Wulf_H._Utian

36. B. Goldacre, *Medical ghostwriters who build a brand*, The Guardian, September 18, 2010, https://www.the-

guardian.com/commentisfree/2010/sep/18/bad-science-medical-ghostwriters, accessed 23 December 2018.

37. N. Singer, *Menopause, as Brought to You by Big Pharma*, New York Times , December 12, 2009, https://www.nytimes.com/2009/12/13/business/13drug.html, accessed 23 December 2018.

38. *ibidem.*

39 A. Kuczynski, *Menopause Forever*, New York Times, June 23, 2002, https://www.nytimes.com/2002/06/23/style/menopause-forever.html, accessed 23 December 2018.

40. E. Wheeler, *Flibanserin: The Female Viagra Is a Failed Me-too Antidepressant*, Mad in America, August 17, 2015, https://www.madinamerica.com/2015/08/flibanserin-the-female-viagra-is-a-failed-me-too-antidepressant/, accessed 23 December 2018.

41. R. Moynihan, *Evening the score on sex drugs: feminist movement or marketing masquerade?*, «British Medical Journal», n. 349, October 17, 2014, p.2

42. *Orgasm Inc.*, Liz Canner, 2009.

43. *66 Peri Menopause / Menopause Symptoms You May Experience Which May Help Some Ladies*, Patient.info, http://patient.info/forums/discuss/66-peri-menopause-menopause-symptoms-you-may-experience-which-may-help-some-ladies-271903, accessed 23 December 2018.

Chapter Two

Menopause is a good thing

1. K. Hawkes, *Grandmothers and Human Evolution*, Margo Wilson Memorial Lecture, McMaster University, Hamilton, October 03, 2013.

2. K. Hawkes, *Grandmas Made Humans Live Longer: Computer Simulation: Chimp Lifespan Evolves Into Human Longevity*, University of Utah News, October 24, 2012, https://archive.unews.utah.edu/news_releases/grandmas-made-humans-live-longer/, accessed 23 December 2018.

3. *ibidem.*

4. K. Hawkes, *Grandmothers and Human Evolution*, Margo Wilson Memorial Lecture, McMaster University, Hamilton, October 03, 2013.

5. J. Oeppen, *Broken Limits to Life Expectancy*, «Science Magazine», vol. 296, n. 5570, 2002, p. 1029-1031

6. K. Hawkes, *Grandmothers and Human Evolution*, Margo Wilson Memorial Lecture, McMaster University, Hamilton, October 03, 2013.

7. *ibidem*.

8. G. Sheehy, *The Silent Passage*, Random House, New York 1991, p. 227.

9. M. Lock, *Encounters with Aging: Mythologies of Menopause in Japan and North America*, University of California Press, Berkley 1993, p. xxvi.

10. J. Colgrove, *The McKeown Thesis: A Historical Controversy and Its Enduring Influence*, «Am J Public Health», vol. 92, n. 5, 2002, p. 725-729.

11. C. Gosden, *Fetal blood chromosome analysis: some new indications for prenatal karyotyping*, Br J Obstet Gynaecol, p. 915-920.

12. K. Hawkes, *Grandmothers and Human Evolution*, Margo Wilson Memorial Lecture, McMaster University, Hamilton, October 03, 2013.

13. F. Marlowe, *The Patriarch Hypothesis : An Alternative Explanation of Menopause*, «Hum Nat.», vol. 11, n. 1, 2000, p. 27-42

14. S. Assari, *Why Do Women Live Longer Than Men?*, World Economic Forum, March 14, 2017, https://www.weforum.org/agenda/2017/03/why-do-women-live-longer-than-men, accessed 23 December 2018.

15. M. Lock, *Encounters with Aging: Mythologies of Menopause in Japan and North America*, University of California Press, Berkeley 1993, p. xxvii.

16. K. Hawkes, *Grandmothers and Human Evolution*, Margo Wilson Memorial Lecture, McMaster University, Hamilton, October 03, 2013.

17. L. Blue, *Why Do Women Live Longer Than Men?*, Time Magazine, August 06, 2008, http://content.time.com/

time/health/article/0,8599,1827162,00.html, accessede 23 December 2018.

18. K. Hawkes, *Grandmothers and Human Evolution*, Margo Wilson Memorial Lecture, McMaster University, Hamilton, October 03, 2013.

19. EG Lufkin, *Estrogen Replacement Therapy for the Prevention of Osteoporosis*, «Am Fam Physician», vol. 40, n. 3, 1989, p.205-212.

20. F. Labrie, *DHEA and the Intracrine Formation of Androgens and Estrogens in Peripheral Target Tissues: Its Role during Aging*, «Steroids», vol. 63, n. 5–6, 1998, p. 322-328

21. K. Hawkes [et al.], *Grandmothering, Menopause, and the Evolution of Human Life Histories*, «PNAS», vol. 95, n. 3, 1998, p. 1337.

22. J. Diamond, *Why Sex is Fun?*, Basic Books, New York 1997.

23. F.S. Vom Saal, *Natural History and Mechanisms of Reproductive Aging in Humans, Laboratory Rodents, and Other Selected Vertebrates*, in AA.VV., *The Physiology of Reproduction*, Raven Press, New York 1994, p. 1213-1313

24. A. Ziomkiewicz, *Evidence for the Cost of Reproduction in Humans: High Lifetime Reproductive Effort Is Associated with Greater Oxidative Stress in Post-Menopausal Women*, PLOS ONE, January 13, 2016, https://journals.plos.org/plosone/article?id=10.1371/journal.pone.0145753, accessed 23 December 2018.

25. E. Yong, *Why Killer Whales (and Humans) Go Through Menopause*, The Atlantic, January 12, 2017, https://www.theatlantic.com/science/archive/2017/01/why-do-killer-whales-go-through-menopause/512783/, accessed 23 December 2018.

26. *ibidem*.

27. *ibidem*.

28. *ibidem*.

29. S. Yin, *Why Do We Inherit Mitochondrial DNA Only From Our Mothers?*, New York Times, June 23, 2016, https://www.nytimes.com/2016/06/24/science/mitochondrial-dna-mothers.html, accessed 23 December 2018.

Chapter Three

Medicine for Menopause

1. A.B. Stockham, *Tokology A Book for Women*, Alice B. Stockholm & Co., Chicago 1889, p. 276
2. *ibidem*, p. 281.
3. Mayo Clinic Staff, *Treatments and Drugs* http://www.mayoclinic.org/diseases-conditions/menopause/basics/treatment/con-20019726
4. Mayo Clinic Staff, Definition, Diseases and Conditions: Menopause, http://www.mayoclinic.org/diseases-conditions/menopause/basics/definition/con-20019726, accessed 23 December 2018.
5. T. Scialli, *Perimenopause: an 'invented' disease*. The Free Library, May 1, 2003, https://www.thefreelibrary.com/Perimenopause%3a+an+%22invented%22+disease.-a0103382411, accessed 23 December 2018.
6. S. Salhan, *Textbook of Gynecology*, Jaypee Brothers Medical Publishers, New Delhi 2012, p. 147.
7. F. Labrie, *Endocrine and Intracrine Sources of Androgens in Women: Inhibition of Breast Cancer and Other Roles of Androgens and Their Precursor Dehydroepiandrosterone* , «Endocrine Reviews», vol. 24, I. 2, 2003, p.156
8. *ibidem*. P.156.
9. J. S. Sandoval-Leon, *Menopause: Changes and Challenges*, Medscape, August 5, 2014, https://reference.medscape.com/features/slideshow/menopause, accessed 23 December 2018.
10. E. Siegal Watkins, *The Estrogen Elixir: A History of Hormone Replacement Therapy in America*, Johns Hopkins University Press, Baltimore 2007, p. 63.
11. N. Kriplen, *The Heroine of the FDA: One woman was all that stood between thalidomide and America*, Discover Magazine 2017, http://discovermagazine.com/2017/march/the-heroine-of-the-fda, accessed 23 December 2018.

12. R. D. Mcfadden, *Frances Oldham Kelsey, Who Saved U.S. Babies From Thalidomide, Dies at 101*, New York Times, August 7, 2015
https://www.nytimes.com/2015/08/08/science/frances-oldham-kelsey-fda-doctor-who-exposed-danger-of-thalidomide-dies-at-101.html?_r=0, accessed 23 December 2018.

13 E. Siegal Watkins, *The Estrogen Elixir: A History of Hormone Replacement Therapy in America*, Johns Hopkins University Press, Baltimore 2007, p. 144.

14. *ibidem*, p. 134.

15. *FDA Denies Employee Harassment Charges*, «Chemical & Engineering News Archive», vol. 52, n. 39, p. 5.

16. E. Siegal Watkins, *The Estrogen Elixir: A History of Hormone Replacement Therapy in America*, Johns Hopkins University Press, Baltimore 2007, p. 136.

17. *ibidem*, p. 139

18. *ibidem*, p. 143

19. *ibidem*, p. 137

20. *ibidem*, p. 140

21. History of the US Food and Drug administration Alexander M Schmidt, taped oral transcript of interview by James Harvey Young, (Chicago Illinois, 1985) p. 40.
https://www.fda.gov/downloads/AboutFDA/WhatWeDo/, accessed 23 December 2018.

22. *ibidem*, p. 43.

23. Wyeth-Ayerst Laboratories Supports Major New Initiative by The American Heart Association Source Wyeth Industries, https://thepharmaletter.com/article/wyeth-ayerst-recalls-redux-and-pondimin
accessed December 23, 2018

24. *Prempro Hormone Replacement Therapy linked to Breast Cancer and Other Serious Health Problems*, Levin Simes LLP, 2014, https://www.levinsimes.com/prempro-hormone-replacement-therapy-linked-to-breast-cancer-and-other-serious-health-problems/, accessed 23 December 2018.

25. *The Experts Do Agree About Hormone Therapy*, The North American Menopause Society, 2017, https://www.-

menopause.org/for-women/menopauseflashes/menopause-symptoms-and-treatments/the-experts-do-agree-about-hormone-therapy, accessed 23 December 2018.

26. *Climacteric*, Home Page, May 3, 2017, http://www.imsociety.org/about_the_journal.php, accessed 23 December 2018.

27. T. Goldberg - B. Fidler, *Conjugated Estrogens/Bazedoxifene (Duavee): A Novel Agent for the Treatment of Moderate-to-Severe Vasomotor Symptoms Associated With Menopause And the Prevention of Postmenopausal Osteoporosis Pharmacy and Therapeutics*, «P&T», vol. 40, n.3, 2015, p.178-182

28. L. Gennari, *Bazedoxifene for the Prevention of Postmenopausal Osteoporosis*, «Therapeutics and Clinical Risk Management», vol. 4, n. 6, 2008, p.1229-1242

29. M. Ratner, *Pfizer reaches out to academia—again*, «Nature Biotechnology Journal», vol. 29, n. 3, 2011, p. 3.

30. E. Palmer, *Duavee: Pfizer is stuck with a hot flash med that took years to get to market*, FierceBiotech, October 3, 2017
http://www.fiercebiotech.com/special-report/duavee-pfizer-stuck-a-hot-flash-med-took-years-to-get-to-market, accessede 23 December 2018.

31. R. M. Lewis, *Endocrine Treatment of Vaginitis of Children and of Women after Menopause*, «Journal of American Medicine», vol. 109, n. 23, 1937, p. 593.

32. *ibidem*. P.593.

33. *ibidem*. p.593.

34. *ibidem*. p.593.

35. K. J. Karnaky, *Uterine Bleeding and Menstruation Its Causes and Treatment, A New Theory*, «Journal of the National Medical Association», vol. xxxii, n. 6, 1940, p. 235-238.

36. B. Seaman, *The Greatest Experiment Ever Performed on Women: Exploding The Estrogen Myth*, Seven Stories Press, New York 2004, p. 37.

37. H. C. Falk, *Atrophic or Senile Vaginitis: Treatment with Dienestrol Cream*, «Journal of the American Geriatric Society», December, 1963, p.1152.

38. G.G. Kuiper, Comparison of the Ligand Binding Specificity and Transcript Tissue Distribution of Estrogen Receptors Alpha and Beta, «Endocrinology», vol. 138, n. 3, 1997, p. 863-870

39. Drugs and Medications, Vagifem Tablet Side Effects, WebMd, http://www.webmd.com/drugs/2/drug-18858-6300/vagifem-tablet/details#side-effects, accessed 23 December 2018.

40. M. L. Krychman, *Vaginal Atrophy: The 21st Century Health Issue Affecting Quality of Life,* Medscape Ob/Gyn, 2007

http://www.medscape.org/viewarticle/561934

41. J. Graedon, *Why is the Cost of Premarin so Outrageous*, The People's Pharmacy, March 21, 2016, https://www.peoplespharmacy.com/2016/03/21/why-is-the-cost-of-premarin-so-outrageous/, accessed 23 December 2018.

42. E. Rosenthal, *As Drug Costs Rise, Bending the Law Is One Remedy*, New York Times, October 22, 2013, https://www.nytimes.com/2013/10/23/health/as-drug-costs-rise-bending-the-law-is-one-remedy.html, accessed 23 December 2018.

43. J. Rosenhek, *Mad with Menopause*, Doctors Review, February 2014, http://www.doctorsreview.com/history/mad-menopause/, accessed 23 December 2018

44. R. Morantz-Sanchez, *Conduct Unbecoming a Woman: Medicine on Trial in Turn-of-the-Century Brooklyn*, Oxford University Press, Oxford 1999, p. 247.

45. *idibem*. P.247

46. J. B. Fleming, *Clitoridectomy -- the disastrous downfall of Isaac Baker Brown*, «The Journal of Obstetrics and Gynaecology of the British Empire», vol. 67, n. 6, 1960, p. 1018.

47. *idibem*. P. 1018

48. E. Siegal Watkins, *The Estrogen Elixir: A History of Hormone Replacement Therapy in America*, Johns Hopkins University Press, Baltimore 2007, p. 62.

49. J. Easton, *Jensen Wins Lasker for Research on Estrogen Receptors*, The University of Chicago Chronicle, vol. 24, n. 2, October 7, 2004, http://chronicle.uchicago.edu/041007/jensen.shtml, accessed 23 December 2018.

50. http://www.bussolasanita.it/schede-1851-menopausa_arriva_il_nuovo_farmaco_per_le_donne_italiane, accessed December 23, 2018.

51. R. S. McIntyre [*et al.*], *Hormone Replacement Therapy and Antidepressant Prescription Patterns: A Reciprocal Relationship*, «Canadian Medical Association Journal», vol. 172, n. 1, 2005, p.57-59.

52. P. Wehrwein, *Astounding increase in antidepressant use by Americans*, Harvard Medical School, October 20, 2011, https://www.health.harvard.edu/blog/astounding-increase-in-antidepressant-use-by-americans-201110203624, accessed 23 December 2018.

53. C. Coupland, *Antidepressant Use and Risk of Suicide and Attempted Suicide or Self Harm in People Aged 20 to 64: Cohort Study Using a Primary Care Database*, theBMJ, 18 February 2015, https://www.bmj.com/content/350/bmj.h517, accessed 23 December 2018.

54. F.J. de Abajo – L.A. García-Rodríguez, *Risk of Upper Gastrointestinal Tract Bleeding Associated with Selective Serotonin Reuptake Inhibitors and Venlafaxine Therapy: Interaction with Nonsteroidal Anti-Inflammatory Drugs and Effect of Acid-Suppressing Agents*, «Arch Gen Psychiatry», vol. 65, n. 7, 2008, p-3-17

55. Y. Sheu [*et al.*], *SSRI Use and Risk of Fractures Among Perimenopausal Women Without Mental Disorders*, «Injury Prevention», vol. 21, n. 6, 2015, p.397-403

56. S. Zoli, *Antidepressivi contro le vampate*, Magazine: Il portale di chi crede nella ricerca, September 9, 2012, http://www.fondazioneveronesi.it/magazine/articoli/ginecologia/antidepressivi-contro-le-vampate accessed 23 December 2018.

57. *ibidem.*

58. W. Duffie, *Deep Dive: ONR-Supported Research Combats Oxygen Toxicity in Navy Divers*, December 8, 2015, https://www.onr.navy.mil/en/Media-Center/Press-Re-

leases/2015/Oxygen-Toxicity-Navy-Divers, accessed 23 December 2018.

59. F. Rosado, *History of Osteoporosis*, Reliawire, June 11, 2007, http://reliawire.com/history-osteoporosis/, accessed 23 December 2018.

60. B. Seaman, *The Greatest Experiment Ever Performed on Women: Exploding The Estrogen Myth*, Seven Stories Press, New York 2004, p. 76.

61. *ibidem*. p. 78.

62. William A. Peck, M.D. RiverVest Investing in Life Science Innovation
https://www.rivervest.com/team/william-a-peck-m-d/ Accessed December 23, 2018.

63. T. Parker-Pope, *The Confusing Diagnosis of Osteopenia*, New York Times, September 7, 2009, https://well.blogs.nytimes.com/2009/09/07/the-confusing-diagnosis-of-osteopenia/, accessed 23 December 2018.

64. K. Murphey, *Splits Form Over How to Address Bone Loss*, New York Times, September 7, 2009, https://www.nytimes.com/2009/09/08/health/08bone.html, accessed 23 December 2018.

65. P. A. Coello, *Drugs for Pre-Osteoporosis: Prevention or Disease Mongering?*, «BMJ», vol. 335, n. 7636, 2008, p. 126-129

66. *Merck's Fosamax Cleared For US Marketing*, thepharmaletter, September 10, 1995, https://www.thepharmaletter.com/article/merck-s-fosamax-cleared-for-us-marketing, accessed 23 December 2018.

67. *ibidem*.

68. S. Kelleher, *Disease Expands Through Marriage of Marketing and Machines*, Seattle Times, June 28, 2005, https://www.seattletimes.com/seattle-news/health/disease-expands-through-marriage-of-marketing-and-machines/, accessed 23 December 2018.

69. *ibidem*.

70. *ibidem*.

71. *ibidem*.

72. S. Boyles, *Drug for Bone Disease Linked to 'Jaw Death'*, WebMD, October 3, 2005, https://www.webmd.com/a-to-z-guides/news/20051003/drug-for-bone-disease-linked-to-jaw-death#1, accessed 23 December 2018.

73. B.A. Lenart - D.G. Lorich - J.M. Lane, *Atypical Fractures of the Femoral Diaphysis in Postmenopausal Women Taking Alendronate*, «New England Journal of Medicine», vol. 358, n. 12, 2008, p.1304-1306.

74. D.M. Black [et al.], *Effects of Continuing or Stopping Alendronate After 5 Years of Treatment: The Fracture Intervention Trial Long-Term Extension (FLEX): A Randomized Trial*, «Journal of the American Medical Association», vol. 296, n. 24, 2006, p.2927-2938.

75. Harvard Women's Health Watch, *What's the story with Fosamax?*, Harvard Health Publishing, November 2008, https://www.health.harvard.edu/diseases-and-conditions/whats_the_story_with_fosamax, accessed 23 December 2018.

76. J.H. Pope [et al.], *Missed Diagnoses of Acute Cardiac Ischemia in the Emergency Department*, «New England Journal of Medicine», vol. 342, n. 16, 2000, p.1163-170

77. L. Kim [et al.], *Sex-Based Disparities in Incidence, Treatment, and Outcomes of Cardiac Arrest in the United States, 2003-2012*, «Journal of the American Heart Association», vol. 5, n. 6, 2016, p. 1-9.

78. C. Wessel Skovlund [et al.], *Association of Hormonal Contraception With Depression*, «Journal of the American Medical Association Psychiatry», vol. 73, n. 11, 2016, p. 1154-1162.

79. D. DeMarco, *New Perspectives on Contraception*, One More Soul, Dayton 1999, p. 18.

80. B. Seaman, *The Doctor's Case Against the Pill*, Hunter House, New York 1995, p.

81. K. Rogers, *How to Stop Your Period*, New York Times, October 18, 2016, https://www.nytimes.com/2016/10/19/well/live/how-to-stop-your-period.html, accessed 23 December 2018.

82. A. Goodnough – K. Zernike, *Seizing on Opioid Crisis, a Drug Maker Lobbies Hard for Its Product*, New York Times,

June 11, 2017, https://www.nytimes.com/2017/06/11/health/vivitrol-drug-opioid-addiction.html, accessed 23 December 2018.

83. M. L. Burstall, *European Policies Influencing Pharmaceutical Innovation*, The National Academy of Sciences, 1991
https://www.ncbi.nlm.nih.gov/books/NBK234307/, accessed 23 December 2018.

84. A. Lapertosa, *Contraccezione, solo il 16 per cento delle italiane usa la pillola: "Come in Iraq"*, Il Fatto Quotidiano, July 2, 2012, http://www.ilfattoquotidiano.it/2012/07/06/contraccezione-solo-16-per-cento-delle-italiane-usa-pillola-come-iraq-e-botswana/254970/, accessed 23 December 2018.

86. *ibidem*.

87. K. O'Grady, *The Female Condom: It's Noisy, It's Ugly and It's Expensive, but It's the Safest Sex Around*, A Friend Indeed, The Free Library, May 1, 2003
https://www.thefreelibrary.com/The+female+condom%3a+it%27s+noisy%2c+it%27s+ugly+and+it%27s+expensive%2c+but+it%27s...-a0103382412, accessed 23 December 2018.

88. L. Iverson, *Drugs: A Very Short Introduction*, Oxford University Press, Oxford 2001, p. 73.

89. S. White Junod – L. Marks, *Women's Trials: The Approval of the First Oral Contraceptive Pill in the United States and Great Britain*, «Journal of the History of Medicine», vol. 57, n. 2, 2002, p. 122.

90. H. M. Behre [*et al.*], *Efficency and Safety of an Injectable Combination Hormonal Contraceptive for Men*, «Journal of Clinical Endocrinology & Metabolism», vol. 101, n. 12, 2016, p. 4779-4788.

91. B. Squires, *The Racist and Sexist History of Keeping Birth Control Side Effects Secret*, Vice, October 17, 2016, https://broadly.vice.com/en_us/article/kzeazz/the-racist-and-sexist-history-of-keeping-birth-control-side-effects-secret, accessed 23 December 2018.

92. D.E. Hoffmann, *The Girl Who Cried Pain: A Bias Against Women in the Treatment of Pain*, «Journal of Law, Medicine & Ethics», vol. 29, n. 1, 2001, p.14.

93. L. Pilote – I. Karp, *GENESIS-PRAXY (GENdEr and Sex determInantS of cardiovascular disease: From bench to beyond-Premature Acute Coronary SYndrome)*, «American Heart Journal», vol. 153, n 5, 2012, p.745.

Chapter Four

The case for diet

1. K. Hawkes, *Grandmothers and Human Evolution*, Margo Wilson Memorial Lecture, McMaster University, Hamilton, October 03, 2013.

2. T. Scott, *America Fooled*, Argo Publishing, Victoria 2006, p. 31.

3. A. Kuczynski, *Menopause Forever*, New York Times, June 23, 2002, https://www.nytimes.com/2002/06/23/style/menopause-forever.html, accessed 23 December 2018.

4. R. Lane, *Adam and Eve Diet*, Hodder Mobius, 2002, p.10

5. V. Korenchevsky [et al.], *The effects of Δ4-androstenedione and Δ5-androstenediol on castrated and ovariectomized rats*, «Biochem», vol. 31, n. 3, 1937, p. 467-474.

6. F. Labrie, *DHEA and the intracrine formation of androgens and estrogens in peripheral target tissues: its role during aging*, «Steroids», vol. 63, n. 5-6, 1998, p.185.

7. J. Cui, *Estrogen Synthesis and Signaling Pathways During Ageing: From Periphery to Brain*, «Trends in Molecular Medicine», vol. 19, n. 3, 2013, p.197.

8. F. Labrie, *DHEA and the intracrine formation of androgens and estrogens in peripheral target tissues: its role during aging*, «Steroids», vol. 63, n. 5-6, 1998, p.

9. Menopause https:/www.mayoclinic.org/diseases-conditions/menopause/symptoms-causes/syc-20353397, accessed December 26, 2018

10. *10 Ways to Deal With Menopause Symptoms*, WebMD, November 10, 2017, https://www.webmd.com/menopause/ss/slideshow-10-ways-to-deal-with-menopause-symptoms, accessed 23 December 2018.

11. L. Cappelloni, *What Are the Symptoms and Signs of Menopause?*, Healthline, July 28, 2016, http://www.healthline.com/health/menopause/symptoms-signs#Overview1, accessed 23 December 2018.

12. J. Thomas, How TV Shows Handle Menopause," slate.com, *February 5, 2013*,
https://slate.com/culture/2013/02/menopause-on-tv-from-the-cosby-show-to-house-of-cards-video.html,
accessed December 26, 2018

13. M. Cimons, *The Medicalization of Menopause- Framing Media Messages In The 20th Century*, University of Maryland Press, Baltimore 2008, p. 31.

14. F.M. Pottenger, *Symptoms of Visceral Disease, a Study of the Vegetative Nervous System in Its Relationship to Clinical Medicine*, C. V. Mosby Company, St. Louis 1919, pp. 248-249.

15. J.P. Pratt [*et al.*], *The Endocrine Treatment of Menopausal Phenomena*, «Journal of the American Medical Association», vol. 109, n. 23, 1937, p,1875-1880

16. D.C. Deecher [*et al.*], *Understanding the Pathophysiology of Vasomotor Symptoms (Hot Flushes and Night Sweats) That Occur in Perimenopause, Menopause, and Postmenopause Life Stages*, «Womens Ment Health», vol. 10, n. 6, 2007, p.247

17. R. Lewis, *Endocrine Treatment of Vaginitis of Children and of Women After Menopause*, «Journal of the American Medical Association», vol. 109, n. 23, 1937, p.593.

18. E. Odeblad [*et al.*], *The Biophysical Properties of the Cervical Vaginal Secretions*, «International Review of Natural Family Planning», vol. 7, n.1, 1983, p.304.

19. E. Odeblad, *Some Notes on the Cervical Crypts*, «Method Research and Reference Centre of Australia», vol, 24, n. 2, 1997, p. 31.

20. *ibidem*.

21. P. Rinck, *Europe celebrates the forgotten pioneer of MRI: Dr. Erik Odeblad*, AuntMinnieEurope.com, June 19, 2012, http://www.auntminnieeurope.com/index.aspx?sec=ser&sub=def&pag=dis&ItemID=606754, accessed 23 December 2018.

22. M. Menárguez [et al.], *Morphological Characterization of Different Human Cervical Mucus Types Using Light and Scanning Electron Microscopy*, «Human Reproduction», vol. 18, n. 9, 2003, p.1782

23. D.J. Portman [et al.], *Genitourinary Syndrome of Menopause: New Terminology for Vulvovaginal Atrophy from the International Society for the Study of Women's Sexual Health and the North American Menopause Society*, «Menopause», vol. 21, n. 10, 2014, p. 1063.

24. L. Dawn [et al.], *Cortisol, Sexual Arousal, and Affect in Response to Sexual Stimuli*, «Journal of Sexual Medicine», vol. 5, n. 9, 2008, p.2111-2118.

25. Mayo Clinic Staff, "Male menopause: Myth or reality?", http://www.mayoclinic.org/healthy-lifestyle/mens-health/in-depth/male-menopause/art-20048056

26. NPR Staff, *Male Birth Control Study Killed After Men Report Side Effects*, NPR, November 2016, http://www.npr.org/sections/health-shots/2016/11/03/500549503/male-birth-control-study-killed-after-men-complain-about-side-effects, accessed 23 December 2018.

27. J. Diamond, *Why Sex Is Fun?*, Basic Books, New York 1997,

28. L. Dawn [et al.], *Cortisol, Sexual Arousal, and Affect in Response to Sexual Stimuli*, «Journal of Sexual Medicine», vol. 5, n. 9, 2008, p.2111-2118.

29. C. Zhao [et al.], *Estrogen receptor β: an overview and update*, «Nuclear Receptor Signaling», vol. 6, n. 003, 2008. p. 1-10

30. J. Cui, *Estrogen Synthesis and Signaling Pathways During Ageing: From Periphery to Brain*, «Trends in Molecular Medicine», vol. 19, n. 3, 2013, p.197209

31. *Estrogen and Women's Emotions*, WebMD, http://www.webmd.com/women/guide/estrogen-and-womens-emotions#1, accessed 23 December 2018.

32. *ibidem*.

33. Amina Zafar, "Estrogen's effects on aging brain explored," CBS News, April 6, 2011 ET

34. J. Jankovic, *Gillian Einstein Leads Research in Women's Brain Health with Inaugural Wilfred and Joyce Posluns Chair*, University of Toronto, March 16, 2017, http://www.dlsph.utoronto.ca/2017/03/gillian-einstein-leads-research-in-womens-brain-health-with-inaugural-wilfred-and-joyce-posluns-chair/, accessed 23 December 2018.

35. J.Q. Zhang, *Distribution and differences of estrogen receptor beta immunoreactivity in the brain of adult male and female rats*, «Brain Research», vol. 935, n. 1-2, 2002, p.73-80

36. *'Brain Fog' of Menopause Confirmed*, University of Rochester Medical Center Newsroom, March 14, 2012, https://www.urmc.rochester.edu/news/story/3436/brain-fog-of-menopause-confirmed.aspx, accessed 23 December 2018.

37. A. Norton, *More Evidence Menopause 'Brain Fog' Is Real*, Healthday News, WebMD, October 12, 2016, http://www.webmd.com/menopause/news/20161012/more-evidence-menopause-brain-fog-is-real#1, accessed 23 December 2018.

38. *ibidem*.

39. A. Norton, HRT Won't Lower Women's Alzheimer's Risk, Healthday News, WebMD, February 16, 2017, https://www.webmd.com/alzheimers/news/20170216/hrt-wont-lower-womens-alzheimers-risk-study-finds#1, accessed 23 December 2018.

40. *ibidem*.

41. *Pfizer signs license deal with UR to develop drug for "hot flashes"*, University of Rochester Medical Center Newsroom, November 1, 2004, https://www.urmc.rochester.edu/news/story/682/pfizer-signs-license-deal-with-ur-to-develop-drug-for-hot-flashes.aspx, accessed 23 December 2018.

42. *Licenses Method of Treatment Patent to Pfizer*, Business Wire, November 1, 2004, https://www.businesswire.-

com/news/home/20041101006013/en/University-Rochester-Licenses-Method-Treatment-Patent-Pfizer, accessed 23 December 2018.

43. ibidem.

44. *The Brain on Menopause*, brainHQ, https://www.brainhq.com/brain-resources/brain-facts-myths/brain-on-menopause, accessed 23 December 2018.

45. ibidem.

46. ibidem.

47. S.N. Nabili, *Insomnia*, eMedicine Health, May 25, 2016, http://www.emedicinehealth.com/insomnia/article_em.htm, accessed 23 December 2018.

48. I. Vargas [et al.], *The Cortisol Awakening Response and Depressive Symptomatology: The Moderating Role of Sleep and Gender*, «Stress Health», vol. 33, n.3, 2017, p.199-210

49. *Giornata mondiale del sonno: l'insonnia cresce tra i giovani*, La Repubblica, March 17, 2016, http://www.repubblica.it/salute/prevenzione/2016/03/17/news/giornata_mondiale_del_sonno-135721349/, accessed 23 December 2018.

50. C. Cirelli, *Sleep and the Price of Plasticity: From Synaptic and Cellular Homeostasis to Memory Consolidation and Integration,* , «Neuron», vol. 81, n.1 , 2014, p.12-34

51. N. Zisapel [et al.], *The relationship between melatonin and cortisol rhythms: clinical implications of melatonin therapy*, «Drug Development Research», vol. 65, n.3, 2005,

52. ibidem.

53. G.J. Elder [et al.], *The cortisol awakening response-- applications and implications for sleep medicine*, «Sleep Medicine Reviews», vol. 18, n. 3, 2014, p.120

54. M. Horsten [et al.], *Depressive symptoms, social support, and lipid profile in healthy middle-aged women*, «Psychosomatic Medicine», vol. 59, n. 5, 1997, p. 527.

55. J. M. Greenblatt, *The Implications of Low Cholesterol in Depression and Suicide*, Mental Disorders, November 16, 2015, https://www.greatplainslaboratory.com/articles-1/2015/11/13/the-implications-of-low-choles-

terol-in-depression-and-suicide, accessed 23 December 2018.

56. H.E. Marano, *The Risks of Low-Fat Diets: A diet low in fat and cholesterol may put you at risk for depression*, Psychology Today, April 29, 2003, https://www.psychologytoday.com/intl/articles/200304/the-risks-low-fat-diets, accessed 23 December 2018.

57. S.R. Davis [et al.], *Understanding weight gain at menopause*, «Climacteric», vol. 15, n. 5, 2012, p.419.

58. *ibidem*.

59. L.M. Brown [et al.], *Central Effects of Estradiol in the Regulation of Adiposity*, «Journal of Steroid Biochemistry and Molecular Biology», vol. 122, n.1-3, 2010, p.68.

60. S. Santosa [et al.], *Adipocyte fatty acid storage factors enhance subcutaneous fat storage in postmenopausal women*, «Diabetes», vol. 62, n. 3, 2013, p-775-782-

61. S.R. Davis [et al.], *Understanding weight gain at menopause*, «Climacteric», vol. 15, n. 5, 2012, p.419.

62. *ibidem*.

63. *Stress May Cause Excess Abdominal Fat in Otherwise Slender Women, Study Conducted at Yale Shows*, Yale News, September 22, 2000, http://news.yale.edu/2000/09/22/stress-may-cause-excess-abdominal-fat-otherwise-slender-women-study-conducted-yale-shows, accessed 23 December 2018.

64. L. Hill, *How important are perky boobs*, Cosmopolitan Magazine, February 26, 2014, http://www.cosmopolitan.com/sex-love/advice/a5734/logan-hill-perky-boobs-advice/, accessed 23 December 2018.

65. E. Narins, *5 Ways to Make Your Chest Look Perkier: And Give Your Bra Some Support*, Cosmopolitan Magazine, August 1, 2016, http://www.cosmopolitan.com/health-fitness/a52435/ways-to-make-your-chest-look-perkier/, accessed 23 December 2018.

66. E. Addley, *'These are just ordinary women' – how breast surgery has soared in the UK*, The Guardian, December 21, 2011, https://www.theguardian.com/society/2011/dec/21/british-women-breast-surgery-rising, accessed 23 December 2018.

67. ibidem.

68. J. Krasny, *Every Parent Should Know The Scandalous History Of Infant Formula*, Business Insider, June 25, 2012, https://www.businessinsider.com/nestles-infant-formula-scandal-2012-6, accessed 23 December 2018.

69. S. Jung [*et al.*], *Dietary Fat Intake During Adolescence and Breast Density Among Young Women*, «Cancer Epidemiology, Biomarkers & Prevention», vol. 25, n. 6, 2016, p. OF1-OF10.

70. C. Nagata [*et al.*], *Association of dietary fat, vegetables and antioxidant micronutrients with skin ageing in Japanese women*, «British Journal of Nutrition», vol. 103, n. 10, 2010, p.1493-1498.

71. *Do Breast Implants Need to Be Replaced Every 10 Years?*, Marketwired, February 12, 2015, http://www.marketwired.com/press-release/do-breast-implants-need-to-be-replaced-every-10-years-1991411.htm, accessed 23 December 2018.

72. R.C. Rabin, *After Mastectomies, an Unexpected Blow: Numb New Breasts*, New York Times, January 29, 2017, https://www.nytimes.com/2017/01/29/well/live/after-mastectomies-an-unexpected-blow-numb-new-breasts.html, accessed 23 December 2018.

73. V. De Falco, *MOC: un esame che misura la salute delle tue ossa*, Menopausa Serena, June 10, 2013, http://menopausaserena.altervista.org/moc-in-menopausa.html, accessed 23 December 2018.

74. *Bone Mineral Screening*, WebMD, October 5, 2016, http://www.webmd.com/menopause/guide/bone-mineral-testing#1, accessed 23 December 2018.

75. E. Villa, *Che cosa è la MOC? Come avviene? Ce lo spiega il Dott. Brambilla*, Humanitas Salute, March 2, 2005, http://www.humanitasalute.it/prima-pagina-ed-eventi/3785-la-moc-contro-losteoporosi/, accessed 23 December 2018.

76. R. Dabirnia [*et al.*], *The relationship between vitamin D receptor (VDR) polymorphism and the occurrence of osteoporosis in menopausal Iranian women*, «Clinical Cases in

Mineral and Bone Metabolism», vol. 13, n.3, 2016, p.190-194.

77. C. Durosier-Izart, *Peripheral skeleton bone strength is positively correlated with total and dairy protein intakes in healthy postmenopausal women*, «American Journal of Clinical Nutrition», vol. 105, n. 2, 2017, p.513.

78. N. Sharma, *Effect of Multiparity and Prolonged Lactation on Bone Mineral Density*, «Journal of Menopausal Medicine», vol. 22, n. 3, 2016, p.161.

79. N.M Al-Daghri, *Inflammation as a contributing factor among postmenopausal Saudi women with osteoporosis*, «Medicine (Baltimore)», vol. 96, n.4, 2017, p. 5.

80. J. Yudkin, *Sweet and Dangerous*, Bantam Books, New York 1973, p. 112.

81. J.L. Saffar [et al.], Osteoporotic effect of a high-carbohydrate diet (Keyes 2000) in golden hamsters, «Archives of Oral Biology», vol. 26, n. 5, 1981, p. 393.

82. A. Shnier [et al.], *Reporting of financial conflicts of interest in clinical practice guidelines: a case study analysis of guidelines from the Canadian Medical Association Infobase*, BMC Health Services Research, 2016, https://bmchealthservres.biomedcentral.com/articles/10.1186/s12913-016-1646-5, accessed 23 December 2018.

83. W. Buchan, *Domestic medicine or a treatise on the prevention and cure of diseases by regimen and simple medicines*, H Chamberlain and others, Dublin, 1772, p. 86.

84. J.E. Manson, *The Latest on Managing Menopausal Symptoms*, Medscape, September 9, 2015, http://www.medscape.com/viewarticle/850583

85. G.P. Chrousos, *Glucocorticoid Therapy and Cushing Syndrome*, Medscape, December 11, 2015, http://emedicine.medscape.com/article/921086-overview#showall, accessed 23 December 2018.

Chapter Five

Fat for balance

1. K. Hawkes [et al.], *Grandmothering, Menopause, and the Evolution of Human Life Histories*, «PNAS», vol. 95, n. 3, 1998, p. 1336-1339.

2. E.A. Schultz – R.H. Lavenda, *The Consequences of Domestication and Sedentism*, in AA.VV. A Perspective on the Human Condition, Oxford University Press, Oxford, 2000, p.196-200

3. A. Huseynova [et al.], *Developmental evidence for obstetric adaptation of the human female pelvis*, «PNAS», vol. 113, n. 19, 2016, p. 5227.

4. A. Mummert [et al.], *Stature and robusticity during the agricultural transition: Evidence from the bioarchaeological record*, «Economics & Human Biology», vol. 9, n. 3, 2011, p.284.

5. C.E. Rossiter – H. Chong, *Relations between maternal height, fetal birthweight and cephalopelvic disproportion suggest that young Nigerian primigravidae grow during pregnancy*, «British Journal of Obstetrics and Gynaecology», vol. 29, n. 5, 1985, p.40.

6. P.M. Catalano [et al.], *Increased fetal adiposity: A very sensitive marker of abnormal in utero development*, «American Journal of Obstetrics and Gynecology», vol. 189, n. 6, 2003, p.1498.

7. University of Colorado Denver, *Early human burials varied widely but most were simple*, ScienceDaily, February 21, 2013, https://www.sciencedaily.com/releases/2013/02/130221084747.htm, accessed 23 December 2018.

8. W. Campbell Douglass, *The Milk Book*, SecondOpinionPublishing, Atlanta 1994, p. 215.

9. S. M. Nelson, *Identity and Subsistence: Gender Strategies for Archaelogy*, Rowan Altamira, Oxford 2007, p. 188.

10. *ibidem*. p. 189.

11. U. Le Guin, *The Space Crone*, in *Dancing at the Edge of the World: Thoughts on Words, Women, Places*, Grove Press, New York 1989, p. 5.

12. F. Labrie [et al.], *DHEA and Its Transformation into Androgen and Estrogens in Peripheral Target Tissues:Intracrinology*, «Frontiers in Neuroendorinology», vol. 22, n.3, 2002, p.156.

13. *ibidem*. p.152.

14. *ibidem*.p 152-182.

15. *ibidem*. p.152-182.

16. E.C. Westman, *Is dietary carbohydrate essential for human nutrition?*, «The American Journal of Clinical Nutrition», vol. 75, n. 5, 2002, p.951-953.

17. R. Lane, *Adam and Eve Diet*, Hodder Mobius, 2002, p.9.

18. P. Gadsby – L. Steele, *The Inuit Paradox. How can people who gorge on fat and rarely see a vegetable be healthier than we are?*, Discover Magazine, October 1, 2004, http://discovermagazine.com/2004/oct/inuit-paradox, accessed 23 December 2018.

19. W.S. McClellan [*et al.*], *Clinical Calorimetry*, in *The Russel Sage Institute of Pathology with the Medical (Cornell) Division of Bellevue Hospital*, New York, 1930, http://www.jbc.org/content/87/3/651.full.pdf

20. R. DuBroff [*et al.*], *Cholesterol confusion and statin controversy*, «World Journal of Cardiology», vol. 7, n. 7, 2015, p.404-409.

21. A. Sekikawa [*et al.*], *Continuous decline in mortality from coronary heart disease in Japan despite a continuous and marked rise in total cholesterol: Japanese experience after the Seven Countries Study*, «International Journal of Epidemiology», vol. 44, n. 5, 2015, p.1614-1624.

22. L. Wroblewski Lissin, *Phytoestrogens and cardiovascular health*, «Journal of the American College of Cardiology», vol. 35, n. 6, 2000, p.1403-1410.

23. R. W. Chesney, *Environmental Factors in Tiny Tim's Near-Fatal Illness*, «Archives of Pediatrics & Adolescent Medicine», vol. 166, n.3, 2012, p.272.

24. Melissa, *What Was Wrong with Tiny Tim?*, Today I Found Out, Feed Your Brain, September 23, 2014, http://www.todayifoundout.com/index.php/2014/09/wrong-tiny-tim/, accessed 23 December 2018.

25. E.M. Brey, *Vascularization: Regenerative Medicine and Tissue Engineering*, CRC Press, Boca Raton 2014, p. 329.

26. D.M. Oh – T.J.- Phillips, *Sex Hormones and Wound Healing*, «Wounds», vol. 18, n. 1, 2006, pp. 8-18.

27. M. Coelho, *Biochemistry of Adipose Tissue: An Endocrine Organ*, «Archives of Medical Science», vol. 9, n. 2, 2013, p.191-200.

28. J.W. Rich-Edwards [*et al.*], *Physical Activity, Body Mass Index, and Ovulatory Disorder*, «Epidemiology», vol. 13, n. 2, 2002, p.184-190.

29. *idibem*.

30. M. Gambarin-Gelwan, *Prevalence of Nonalcoholic Fatty Liver Disease in Women With Polycystic Ovary Syndrome*, «Clinical gastroenterology and Hepatology», vol. 5, n. 4, 2007, p.496-501.

ABOUT THE AUTHOR

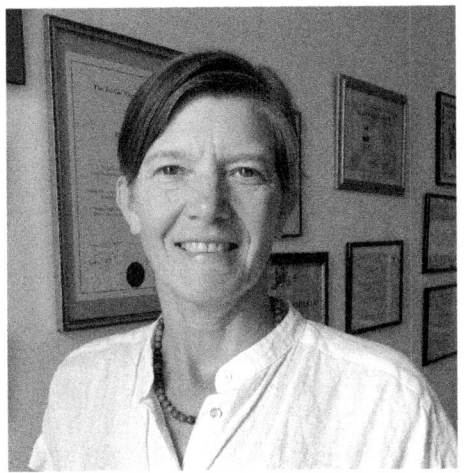

Elizabeth Bright ND, DO, (New York 1963) is an American Naturopath and Osteopath practicing in Genova and Milan, Italy. She lived in China where she learned traditional Chinese medicine and traditional Kung Fu, She became a master of Chau Ka Kung Fu in 2004. She speaks several languages. She founded two organic restaurants in Washington, D.C. where she was chef-owner. She is co-author of The Science of Ageing Backward: Re-generation-X